CHEMOTHERAPY OF
GYNAECOLOGICAL MALIGNANCIES

CHEMOTHERAPY OF GYNAECOLOGICAL MALIGNANCIES

GRAHAM H. BARKER, MB, BS, FRCS(Ed), MRCOG

Senior Registrar in Obstetrics and Gynaecology,
Middlesex and Central Middlesex Hospitals, London.
Formerly Lecturer, Institute of Cancer Research,
and Registrar at the Royal Marsden Hospital,
Chelsea Hospital for Women,
and Queen Charlotte's Hospital, London.

 CASTLE HOUSE PUBLICATIONS LTD

First published 1983 by
Castle House Publications Ltd
Castle House, 27 London Road
Tunbridge Wells, Kent

British Cataloguing in Publication Data
Barker, Graham H.
    Chemotherapy of gynaecological malignancies
    1. Cancer—Chemotherapy
    I. Title
    616.99′4061   RC271.C5

ISBN 0-7194-0082-1

Typeset in Linoterm Times by
Keyset Composition, Colchester

Printed and bound in Great Britain by
Biddles Ltd, Guildford and King's Lynn

Contents

Preface

The recent and rapid development of interest in the chemotherapy of gynaecological cancer has created a need for a comprehensive account of our present knowledge. What was conceived as a short introduction to the subject has grown into a record of the current state of the art to date and, I hope, a source of reference.

Fortunately I have been regularly invited to lecture on the MRCOG Part I and Part II examinations revision courses held at Queen Charlotte's, Hammersmith and King's College Hospitals, London, and these lectures formed the origins of this book. The first half covers the MRCOG Part I requirements (and beyond) concerning the basic pharmacology of antimitotic drugs, and the second half covers the Part II clinical applications. However, the principal aim of this book is to present the subject in depth to oncologists who are not gynaecologists, and to gynaecologists who are not primarily oncologists.

I have reluctantly refrained from indulging in a large introductory chapter on the history of these fascinating drugs but have not lost the opportunity of inserting, via references, a hint or two of the historical circumstances surrounding the treatment development of these malignancies within the text of each chapter.

During the preparation of this book I have received many helpful answers to my enquiries. In particular I would like to record my appreciation of the following people who have kindly provided me with information: Dr Ray Burnett and the staff of Leo Laboratories Ltd, Doreen Perks and the staff of Bristol Myers Oncology Ltd, Dr Tal Latief of the Queen Elizabeth Hospital, Birmingham, Dr Adrian Jones and Dr Shanti Raju of the Royal Marsden Hospitals, London and Surrey, Mr Nick Siddle of the King's College Hospital MRCOG revision course, Drs Rob Buckman and Gordon Rustin of the London Oncology Club and the staffs of the libraries of the Chester Beatty Research Institute of the Institute of Cancer Research, London, the Institute of Obstetrics and Gynaecology, Queen Charlotte's Hospital, London, and the Royal College of Obstetrics and Gynaecology. I would also like to express my gratitude to Mrs Wendy Hunter and Mr Donald Reinders of Castle House Publications Ltd, editor Caroline Richmond, and to my wife, Esther, for all their assistance and encouragement.

Fundamentally this text bears witness to the great debt I owe to Dr Eve Wiltshaw who, having helped pioneer cancer chemotherapy in the United States and the United Kingdom from its tentative early days to its present position as an established cancer treatment modality, found time to take a young gynaecologist into her unit and shared with him the benefits of her extensive experience, her philosophies concerning the application of chemotherapy by the most efficient means, her strict criteria for the assessment of response and, above all, her driving desire to seek improvements constantly in the treatment offered. The young gynaecologist was fascinated and inspired to share with others, via these pages, this knowledge and understanding of cancer chemotherapy as applied to gynaecology.

The overall treatment of gynaecological cancers is a partial success story with some major triumphs and many dismal failures. We can rejoice in the knowledge that at the present time about half our patients with gynaecological malignancies are cured but we must now concentrate upon the other half. The basic processes of cancer surgery and radiotherapy have not altered a great deal in the last fifty years and early diagnosis programmes are yet to be fully exploited. Cancer chemotherapy, however, is developing rapidly both in the number and variety of agents available and in the techniques by which they are administered. Many now feel that it is in this direction that further interest should be turned in an effort to help that other half of women whose lives are untimely ended by malignant disease of their reproductive organs.

Graham H. Barker
London, 1983

Chapter One

Use of Cytotoxic Agents

Before offering any form of anticancer treatment—surgery, radiotherapy, chemotherapy, immunotherapy—the aims of the treatment should be clearly borne in mind. Is the treatment to be curative, adjunctive and preventative, or palliative? All forms of anticancer treatments are expensive, and frequently create for the patient inconvenience and the risk of side effects, morbidity and even mortality. Indiscriminate use of any anticancer modality is therefore to be deprecated.

Surgery is frequently the method of diagnosis and the initial form of therapy. Surgery should be radical only when it is likely to be beneficial. Before the advent of chemotherapy the only additional therapy for cancer was various forms of irradiation, which can often produce short- and long-term side effects, toxicity and considerable morbidity. Efforts have been made recently to evaluate the benefits or otherwise of radiotherapy in a variety of malignant conditions. In some, such as cervical carcinoma and dysgerminoma of the ovary, it has an undoubted role, but in other tumour states radiotherapy may be damaging and produce no treatment advantage for the patient.

The same must be said for chemotherapy—patients should not receive drugs without some hope of benefit and if chemotherapy is clearly not fulfilling this aim in a particular patient it should be withdrawn.

There is no real comfort for a patient to receive a drug which she and her doctor both know is showing no benefit and eventually it undermines the faith a patient has in her doctor's judgement. It is far better to discontinue useless therapy and contemplate either new treatment or stop treatment in favour of supportive and analgesic care.

For many stages, grades and types of tumour, chemotherapy offers clear and documented benefits for the patient, but in others chemotherapy might be given in the hope of improving the patient's situation; whilst all would agree that the best form of palliation is cure, it is well established that beneficial effects such as prolonged survival, and relief of pain, may be obtained from chemotherapy which will not, in fact, be curative.

Before chemotherapeutic agents are used for palliation two factors should be carefully considered: 1) if survival cannot be prolonged and therapy is mainly for the relief of symptoms such as pain, are there any other forms of analgesia, eg

1

regional blockade, which are more effective and less toxic? Morphine is obviously preferable to Adriamycin in this context, and cheaper too; 2) is chemotherapy being given as psychological support for the patient (and her doctors) to ameliorate an essentially hopeless situation by injecting, literally, false hope?

Lathrop and Frates (1980) for example have reported that 62 patients with intractable pelvic pain secondary to pelvic malignancy were treated with percutaneous retrograde arterial infusion of nitrogen mustard. Fifty-six patients experienced excellent or good pain relief with documented improvement of physical performance.

The balance between interfering with the quality of a patient's life and the expected benefit from chemotherapy may be altered in various situations. Some primary cancers, for example trophoblastic disease, can be successfully treated with chemotherapy, and the temporary reduction in the quality of life for that patient is completely justified. The same aggressive chemotherapy might not be appropriate in a terminal care setting where drugs may well be given, third or fourth line, with little hope of anything more than a small chance of remission.

With more understanding of multimodal treatment of malignancies, it is hoped that chemotherapy will be given at the appropriate time in the management, and not relegated to some sort of salvage role when the patient is moribund from failed surgery and failed radiotherapy. With a thorough knowledge of the potential of modern agents clinicians can judge with accuracy the expected benefit in each case—and many patients who appear to be 'too ill for chemotherapy' after presenting late, or following debilitating surgery, will, in fact, with correct treatment, respond and recover remarkably well. This sort of expertise and judgement is acquired by those who use chemotherapy frequently and see many cases referred to them, and, of course, know the potential and limitations of the agents involved.

Quality of life

Newton (1979) found it difficult to classify the quality of life for gynaecological oncology patients but divided it into body functions, work and activity, and family relationships—to which the Karnofsky assessment attaches a score—see Chapter 3. It would seem that an appropriate aim of therapy would be to restore these basic components of life, with a reasonable prospect of longevity, to the state before the cancer was diagnosed. This may be difficult in that the patient's life hitherto may be perceived differently which, as Newton states, 'adds a new and usually unpleasant dimension to an individual's concept of the good life'. Assessment of life quality, and a patient's expectations thereof, by the clinician, may be difficult—Kuebler-Ross (1969) has outlined the types of response patients are likely to produce—denial, anger, bargaining, depression, resignation—and this may modify the expected life quality and the effects of therapy considerably.

Chemotherapy and terminal care

As in the cases of Lathrops and Frates (1980), there may be defined roles for chemotherapy to assist in the management of the end stage patient. However, the side effects of treatment must be taken into consideration before attempts to produce analgesia in this manner are made, or indeed by any manner—intrathecal injections, spinal cordotomies, regional blockades, intramuscular injections of narcotics, narcotic suppositories, etc. However, some would see terminal care as the removal and protection of patients from 'the high technology, cure orientated care of patients in hospitals' (Doyle 1981) and placing them in hospices and the like where the staff devote their energies to palliation and the provision of emotional contentment and spiritual peace.

Long-term hope

It should be remembered, however, that many useful phase I studies of new anticancer drugs are performed on patients with end stage disease, yielding valuable information. Imaginative use of cytotoxic agents under strict trial, and occasionally serendipitous, conditions has led to the formation of highly useful combinations, eg vincristine, actinomycin D, cyclophosphamide, and cisplatin, bleomycin and vinblastine. This does not mean that every patient should be constantly bombarded with a variety of chemotherapeutic agents until death. One or two cancer treatment centres have given no service to chemotherapy by offering unpleasant regimens to terminal patients until the very day of death. Nevertheless, hope can be an important ingredient in the care of cancer patients and many patients, of all ages, are anxious to try new compounds or combinations and persevere with whatever side effects may be encountered.

Ideally all patients who receive any anticancer treatment modality should be recorded and the benefit, if any, of say radiotherapy or chemotherapy be calculated and combined in a series. Therefore, although a patient's tumour may have shown no response to a particular regimen this should be recorded and collated into meaningful data which will prove helpful to other workers. Very often complacency, or conversely excessive despair, exists in a unit unnecessarily if that unit is not constantly calculating and contemplating the results of its cancer treatments. Familiarity with trials already recorded in the literature will allow some patients to benefit from known activity in second and third line treatments and also prevent other patients from treatment already demonstrated, by other units, to be useless.

Cost and benefit

Some might argue that since the majority of cancers affect the relatively elderly population there is little economic sense in spending large sums of money upon the research, development and use of anticancer therapies. Others regard the treatment of cancer as a biological problem which must be faced and overcome. Since hospital drug costs are easily calculated, that spent on anticancer chemotherapy, in particular, may be identified and criticised. Individual drug therapy programmes may be readily costed and attacks made upon their economic validity. However, the other two main anticancer treatment modalities—surgery and radiotherapy—are also expensive, but their cost in real terms, including theatre and machine time, inpatient time etc., is more difficult to calculate.

Bush (1979) for example estimated that the direct cost of treatment per patient for carcinoma of the cervix with radiotherapy in Toronto in 1976 was about $3,000. In examining the retail cost of drugs in a chemotherapy programme one sees, in part, some of the colossal research and development costs required to introduce and sustain a new drug (of whatever use) in the pharmaceutical market of today. These costs vary greatly from drug to drug; a typical list for patients in 1979 included 500 mg 5 fluorouracil as $1.55 compared to Adriamycin 50 mg as $75.00 (Glascoe 1979). In assessing the cost of surgery the cost of the hospital bed must be taken into account and an average cost per day in 1979 was around $400 (Glascoe 1979). One can imagine that any new drug which is effective, and had passed through about ten years of trials before reaching the market, is unlikely to be costed at a few dollars per kilo!

In a detailed cost-benefit analysis of cancer chemotherapy in a Swedish hospital Mattson et al. (1979) found that the use of chemotherapy for advanced malignant disease increased from a few per cent in 1973 to 60% during 1977 corresponding to an increase in the cost of drugs from $10,000 to $200,000, but even this figure was still less than 3% of the medical budget. They emphasised the treatment aim of getting patients back to a life which was as normal as possible, including a return to work, living as much as possible in their own homes. They calculated that through improvements of performance obtained by chemotherapy, most patients could lead their lives in their own environment giving more patients an opportunity to receive anticancer chemotherapy in limited resources, and in their department by applying chemotherapy the number of treated patients increased in excess of 50% without any increases in resources, ie from 317 to 488. They concluded that since more than 90% of their medical budget consists, as in most institutions, of salary and maintenance costs, which are relatively static whatever the number of patients treated, the increase in those numbers treated effectively creates cheaper medical care, but, above all, the survival rate and the quality of life for many of their patients were improved.

In England and Wales three out of every ten people develop cancer but 31% of men and 43% of women are still alive five years after diagnosis. In 1976 the total cost of cancer care was thought to be £250,000,000, equivalent to 5% of the total National Health Service costs, or 15% of the cost of acute services. The 1979 estimate is thought to be nearer £300–£400,000,000. The charitable and Government funded research organisations spend some £40,000,000 on research per annum (Report of the Advisory Committee on Cancer Registration from the Office of Population Censuses and Surveys 1982).

In his discussion on the risk/benefit ratios in the management of gynaecological cancer, Morris (1981) emphasises that the optimum in patient care is best achieved by individualisation with proper selection of the specific treatment for each patient and for the particular lesion, with joint appraisal by experts of each anticancer treatment modality—the decision should be to employ the least radical procedure possible for the individual case, keeping cost, hospitalisation, risk of injury or complication to a minimum, and still offer the maximum statistical chance of cure, prolonged survival and improvement in the quality of life.

References

Bush, R. S., Malignancies of the ovary, uterus and cervix. *Edward Arnold*, 1979, p. 19.

Doyle, D., Hospice care. *Update*, Dec. 1st 1981, 1637–1642.

Glascoe, S., American health care—how the system doesn't work. *World Medicine*, 1979, Nov. 17th, p. 49.

Kuebler-Ross, E., *Death and dying*, Toronto, 1969, Macmillan.

Lathrop, J. C., Frates, R. E., Arterial infusion of nitrogen mustard in the treatment of intractable pelvic pain of malignant origin. *Cancer*, 1980, **45**, 432–8.

Mattson, W., Gynning, I., Carlsson B., Mauritzon, S.-E., Cancer chemotherapy in advanced malignant disease. A cost benefit analysis. *Acta Radiologica Oncology*, 1979, **18**, 509.

Morris, J. M., Risk/benefit ratios in the management of gynecologic cancer. *Cancer*, 1981, **48**, 642–9.

Newton, M., Quality of life for the gynecologic oncology patient. *Am. J. Obstet. Gynecol.*, 1979, **134**, 866.

Report of the Advisory Committee on Cancer Registration, *Cancer Registration in the 1980s* (series MBl no 6), London, HMSO, 1982.

Chapter Two

Aspects of Tumour Growth

Cell kinetics

Although we accept that a tumour represents a disturbance in the normal construction of tissues, it is naïve to regard it as a wild and unrestricted growth. Studies of cell kinetics reveal that tumour growth may occur as a result of a decrease in cell death as well as increased cell proliferation. Although mitotic rates (*mitotic index* = number of mitoses per 100 cells) have traditionally been taken as of prognostic value, they yield relatively little information about tumour growth.

Studies such as those involving the use of tritiated thymidine (Taylor 1957) gave the first indication that DNA (deoxyribonucleic acid) synthesis takes place only during one small part of its life cycle. Furthermore, each tumour may exhibit variable growth patterns and, within a tumour, different parts may show differential growth. This occurs by variations in intermitotic times, and in the proportion of cells that are in the proliferative phase of the cycle; the latter is known as the *growth fraction*.

Mitosis is often referred to as the M phase of the cell cycle. Cell metabolism then follows with no attempt at further replication ie the G_1 first post-mitotic gap phase—see Figure 2.1. DNA synthesis then occurs ie the S phase, leading to the M phase again. The cell cycle may frequently stop (G_0 phase); cells of normal tissues replicate only under special circumstances, eg healing after injury.

Tumour cells may thus be in several states: preparing for replication, replicating or resting. This was first recognised by Mendelsohn (1960). Most cytotoxic therapy is only effective during the first two states ie the M and G_1 phases— unfortunately, the cells to be attacked spend most of their time in the resting state.

Classification of cytotoxic agents

Bruce et al. (1966) classified cytotoxic agents according to their effects on two mouse cell systems—the marrow stem cell and the mouse lymphoma cells. The effectiveness of various drugs was measured by comparison of their effects on cells with varying cell generation times and higher growth fractions. Drugs can be divided simply into non phase-specific agents which can attack cells in any phase of

6

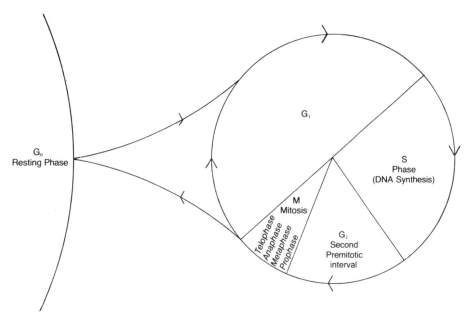

Fig. 2.1 The cell cycle—some authorities consider that cells in G_0 and G_1 are in the same state.

the cell cycle, eg alkylating agents, antitumour antibiotics, cisplatin; and phase-specific agents, eg M phase drugs—vincristine and vinblastine; and S phase drugs—methotrexate, hydroxyurea. Phase-specific drugs are only or mainly effective at a certain phase in the cell cycle.

Cell cycle time

The cell cycle time is the time between successive cell divisions and can be measured using radioactive labelling techniques. Denekemp and Fowler (1977) showed that the normal cell cycle time of normal rabbit skin was 125–750 hours, while that of rabbit skin tumour was a mere 21 hours. Similarly, normal human cervix cells divide every 100–600 hours, but tumour cells divide every 15 hours.

If the interval between cell divisions is constant, then the cell population will double its size at regular intervals and produce exponential growth. Tumours usually show exponential growth when they are small, but usually the time to double the tumour volume (*doubling time*) increases with tumour size. The reason that doubling times usually exceed, therefore, the median cell cycle time is that many cells in the tumour population are not proliferating, and some cells die and are eliminated from the tumour mass.

Tumour characteristics

It is difficult to compare tumours of laboratory animals with those of humans. In general, mouse tumours grow about 30 times faster than human tumours and this, of course, is paralleled by their relative life spans. Nevertheless, regardless of species, it is the physical environment of the tumour that is important to tumour growth and therapy. Although the maximum diffusion distances for nutrients, according to Fowler and Denekemp (1979) are different in human and mouse tumours, the proportion of hypoxic cells is the same, and is of therapeutic significance.

Therapeutic ratio

Cytotoxic drugs are transported by the blood to tumour cells. The vascular supply of tumour cells is less than that of normal tissues; also the majority of the tumour cells are not proliferating. To complicate matters, many normal cells are fast replicating, eg gut lining, hair follicles, bone marrow, and may suffer more than the tumour cells.The concept of the *therapeutic ratio*—the effect on the tumour relative to that on the normal tissue—becomes important, not only in chemotherapy but also in radiotherapy, where fractionation of treatment mirrors repeated chemotherapeutic attack over short intervals with cycle and phase specific drugs.

According to the first law of cell kinetics, in response to a single dose of chemotherapy a certain proportion of cells are killed, not a certain number. *Cell kill* is usually expressed as a logarithm—*log kill*.

Clonogenicity

Many clinicians have regarded tumour cells as one regards weeds in a garden—if the seeds land on normal tissue a cancer will grow. However, this concept is misleading. Laboratory workers who try to grow human cancer cells in vitro or in animal xenograft experiments know the difficulties of getting tumours to thrive, not the least of which is that a tumour mass needs to be of a certain minimum number of cells to survive. Cancer cells appear to live in symbiotic clumps and can be exceedingly difficult to culture.

The biology of metastases is complex. Other explanations may be advanced to account for 'seeding'. For example, vaginal vault recurrence of endometrial carcinoma treated by hysterectomy is fairly common (see Chapter 17) and its incidence can be reduced by preoperative or postoperative radiotherapy to the vault. It would therefore seem likely that because preoperative treatment is beneficial, vault recurrence is possibly due to existing subepithelial lymphatic invasion at the time of surgery, rather than to cancer cells dropping out of the cervix and implanting in the relatively hostile vaginal environment. It might help to explain why aspirates of tumours such as mammary carcinoma taken with fine needles do not leave a track or skin deposits behind them while thick needle biopsies may do so.

Furthermore, it is apparent that only a few of the cells in any given tumour are clonogenic, ie capable of producing a new tumour if they survive in the same or new location. They are analogous to bone marrow, in which only the stem cells are capable of regeneration. Many cells of a tumour, therefore, are destined to be *end cells*—incapable of regeneration or metastasis.

The cell kinetics of *total* cell populations give no indication of the clonogenic potential of the tumour cells. Cell kinetics are based on the whole tumour, but curability depends on the proportion and characteristics of the clonogenic cells. This puts a major limitation on attempts to apply cell kinetics to chemotherapy, or, indeed, to radiotherapy. However, even if a clonogenic cell separates from the main tumour mass it may only produce maturing end cells and not a metastasis. This partly explains the histopathological description of 'differentiation' and degrees of malignancy. Well-differentiated malignant ovarian cysts presumably containing few clonogenic cells may not disseminate on rupture at surgery, whereas others, less well differentiated, invariably do.

Recurrences of tumours some years after initial treatment may be the result of growth from a very small number of surviving cells which are clonogenic, and, of course, relapses may occur earlier if doubling times are short. Cancer treatment of all modalities—surgery, radiotherapy and chemotherapy—is aimed at eradicating all clonogenic cells in the shortest possible time.

References

Bruce, W. R., Meaker, B. E., Valeriote, F. A., Comparison of the sensitivity of normal haematopoetic and transplanted lymphoma colony forming cells to chemotherapeutic agents administered in vivo. *Proc. Natl. Cancer Inst.*, 1966, **37**, 233–45.

Denekemp, J., Fowler, J. F., in *Cancer: a Comprehensive Treatise*, Vol. 6, edited by Becker, F. F., Plenum, New York and London, 1977.

Fowler, J. F., Denekemp, J., A review of hypoxic cell radiosensitisation in experimental tumours. *Pharmacology and Therapeutics*, 1979, **7**, 413.

Mendelsohn, M. L., *Science*, 1960, **132**, 1496.

Taylor, J. H., Woods, P. S., Hughes, W. L., The organisation and duplication of chromosomes as revealed by autoradiographic studies using tritium labelled thymidine. *Proc. Natl. Acad. Sci.*, 1957, **43**, 122.

Chapter Three

Therapeutic Strategy

Methods of attack

There have been, and still are, many attempts to utilise knowledge of cell kinetics and drug specificity in scheduling chemotherapeutic treatment of various cancers. These synchronisation attempts have not been very successful clinically, despite their scientific appeal.

It is, for example, popular in these scheduled drug regimens to give a spindle poison, such as vinblastine, in an attempt to arrest as many cells as possible in the M phase. As the drug is metabolised and excreted, after several hours its concentration starts to fall. This allows the backlog of arrested tumour cells to move forward *en masse*, to be attacked as one by the injection of another phase specific drug. To this sequence can be added a cycle phase nonspecific drug such as an alkylating agent or antitumour antibiotic such as doxorubicin (Adriamycin) to inhibit cells that are not synchronised. For good measure, a drug like methotrexate which has a long half life, able to sustain reasonable blood and tissue levels for a prolonged period, is added in order to attack the stragglers. The idea is appealing.

There are many reasons for the failure of this approach. Firstly, not all the cells have the same kinetics, as mentioned earlier. Secondly, the tumour will recur unless all the clonogenic cells are destroyed, and the kinetics of the clonogenic cells may well vary from the rest. Thirdly, important normal cells, such as those in the bone marrow, may well be synchronised and then eliminated with the tumour.

Metabolism and excretion

Some drugs require activation before they become cytotoxic, and most are excreted relatively quickly from the body via the kidneys or liver. This rapid excretion prevents excessive toxicity in many cases and this fact can be used to advantage in autologous marrow grafting (see Chapter 22).

Cyclophosphamide, for example, has a plasma half life of about six hours (Bagley et al. 1973); Dr Tom Connors and his associates (1974) in the MRC Toxicology Unit at Carshalton, England, have shown that the liver converts the inactive cyclophosphamide to 4-hydroxycyclophosphamide through to phosphoramide mustard, which is cytotoxic. 6-Mercaptopurine, used in the treatment of acute leukaemia, has a half life following intravenous injection of 47 minutes in adults and only 21 minutes in children (Loo et al. 1968).

Methotrexate, for example, is excreted almost entirely via the kidney unmetabolised. However, the rate of excretion can be slow compared with, say, cyclophosphamide, with high plasma levels lasting several days and total excretion incomplete after several weeks especially if renal function is impaired. Chances of developing toxic effects are therefore high and folinic acid rescue may be required if large doses are left to circulate for long periods in the body.

Routes of administration and distribution

Not all cytotoxic agents can even partially be absorbed by the intestinal tract. Some cause nausea and their total gut absorption will be reduced if some of the dose is vomited. For these reasons, many cytotoxic agents are administered by intravenous injection. Small doses of, for example, methotrexate, chlorambucil, and cyclophosphamide may be given orally, but drugs like doxorubicin can only be given intravenously.

This also raises the question of patient compliance. Many clinicians are happier to administer drugs parenterally to ensure that the patient receives them, rather than rely upon patient compliance, which is notoriously poor in other fields of drug therapy. Few patients are going to admit to their oncologist that they have not been taking their medication given for cancer even if they have been putting the tablets down the toilet rather than experience unpleasant side effects such as nausea.

Although the blood carries the drugs to all parts of the body, some areas have a poor vascular supply, and target organ uptake may vary. An example of this is the poor entrance of methotrexate into cerebrospinal fluid, making intrathecal administration necessary in some cancer treatments where the central nervous system may be involved. On the other hand, 5-fluorouracil is an example of a drug which is distributed well, including concentrating in the cerebrospinal fluid.

Scheduling

Leaving aside the dubious advantage of kinetic orientated drug administration, most chemotherapy regimens involve the administrations of repeated doses at set time intervals, eg weekly or monthly. Just as with the fractionation of radiotherapy treatments, the time interval between injections of chemotherapeutic agents allows normal cells—especially those of the bone marrow—to recover and replenish, while it is hoped that although tumour cells also recover during the interval, they will do so in progressively reduced numbers (see Figure 3.1).

In the past the choice of interval between 'pulses' of chemotherapy has been somewhat arbitrary, often a combination of marrow function recovery time and hospital administrative convenience, eg a month. Recently some clinicians have questioned this and are now giving chemotherapy based upon individual recovery periods. Thus if patient X has marrow recovery after 19 days she or he should be

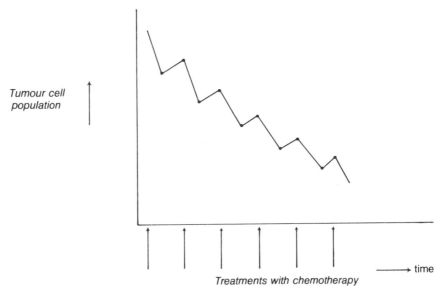

Tumour cell
population

Treatments with chemotherapy

Fig. 3.1   Decline in tumour cell population during chemotherapy

given the next course of chemotherapy then, and not wait for the same time interval as patient Y with a 31-day recovery time. The trend now is towards higher-dose chemotherapy keeping the pulse interval (between courses) as short as is safely possible, in order to prevent excessive tumour recovery.

Single or multiple agent therapy?

It should be remembered that cancer chemotherapy emerged at about the same time as the chemotherapy of tuberculosis: each of the early antituberculous drugs, such as streptomycin, could reduce the bacterial population but not totally eradicate it. However, total cures were obtained when the drugs were given in combination. The extrapolation to cancer chemotherapy was easy to make. However, multiple drugs of the same type used together, eg three alkylating agents, increased toxicity but not efficacy. Combinations of cytotoxic drugs now are mostly chosen for their ability to attack different parts and mechanisms of the reproducing cancer cell at different parts of the cycle. Obviously the addition of each drug increases toxicity and possible side effects.

There may have been a tendency in the past to add agents on theoretical grounds without there being a clear advantage to the patient in terms of remission or survival. At the Royal Marsden Hospital we could not, for example, demonstrate that the addition of doxorubicin (Adriamycin) to low dose cisplatin and chlorambucil did very much, if anything, to improve the remission rate or survival of patients with advanced ovarian carcinoma (Barker and Wiltshaw 1981). Doxorubicin did, however, increase the side effects (alopecia), toxicity (cardiac), and cost. However, by sensible selection, and adequate phase II and phase III (see Chapter 4) trials, the most efficacious combinations can be selected.

Continuous therapy

It was popular for gynaecologists to administer cytotoxic agents such as oral alkylating agents, eg chlorambucil, treosulphan, in small doses on a continuous daily basis. The disadvantage of this is that the dose is often insufficient, and may give rise to the development of acute myeloblastic leukaemia which is refractory to treatment. Reimer et al. (1977) reported 13 patients who developed acute leukaemia out of 5455 with advanced ovarian carcinoma. Six alkylating agents (thiotepa, uracil mustard, cyclophosphamide, melphalan, chlorambucil, hexamethylmelamine) were involved with a median treatment duration of 19 months. Einhorn (1978) reported four leukaemia cases out of 48 patients surviving over three years who had received at least 300 mg of melphalan; those developing acute leukaemia had received 800 mg or more. Significantly, Fennelly in 1982 compared his regimen of intermittent treosulphan, with no development of leukaemia in 100 patients, to that of continuous treosulphan by Pederson-Bjergaard et al. (1980), who reported eight cases out of 553; six of the eight had been on continuous treosulphan for two more years. It is a tragedy to have been cured of ovarian cancer, or at least be in good remission from the tumour, only to succumb to drug-induced leukaemia. Giving intermittent doses of oral alkylating agents for, say, two weeks out of every four virtually eliminates the leukaemia risk. One should also remember that host immune defences, which are probably vital to the success of cancer therapy, are also suppressed by chemotherapy and must also have time to recover.

When to stop therapy

If a solid tumour is sensitive to chemotherapy it will shrink, but, even though it disappears clinically, an undetectable tumour may still have 10^6 viable cells remaining. A patient close to death with an advanced tumour may have 10^{12} tumour cells (Frei 1972). Assuming that chemotherapy removes 99.9% of tumour cells, then 10^9 cells would remain; and even if further chemotherapy removed 99.999% of these cells, assuming no further cell loss, it would only take 16.7 doubling times to recreate the original tumour.

In dealing with leukaemia, for instance, duration of treatment can be geared to the disappearance of leukaemia cells in the bloodstream and bone marrow. The total disappearance of a solid tumour is more difficult to assess. The disappearance of macroscopic tumour may leave microscopic tumours which may contain clonogenic cells capable of recurrence, possibly some considerable time later.

The optimum time for discontinuing therapy cannot be given with certainty for any patient. Obviously clinicians must make every effort to confirm that the disease has been eradicated before stopping chemotherapy. Some advocate small 'maintenance' doses for the rest of the patient's life in some cases, eg alkylating agents in ovarian cancer, but there is little evidence to suggest that late recurrences are prevented this way, and the resulting marrow suppression may prejudice further chemotherapy if the disease recurs while on treatment.

However, since the mid 1970s there has been a trend towards giving high dose combination chemotherapy in short pulses for a wide variety of solid tumours, eg testicular teratoma, and this is proving more effective than prolonged low dose drug administration. Occasionally the toxicity of such regimens proves to be the deciding factor in when to stop therapy.

The use of a 'second look' operation such as laparoscopy and laparotomy is being evaluated as a means of deciding when therapy can be discontinued. However, even when peritoneal washings and multiple biopsies are negative, and the patient is thought to be tumour-free, late recurrences of, for example, ovarian cancer have been found (see Chapter 10). Before therapy is discontinued every effort must be made to evaluate the possibility of residual tumour; avoid setting arbitrary time limits based on little, if any, cogent data.

Effects of surgery and radiotherapy

After the destruction or removal of large tumours by surgery or radiation, some of the remaining tumour cells may be stimulated to enter the active part of the cell cycle, and this renders them more susceptible to chemotherapeutic or radio-therapeutic attack. This has been referred to as *recruitment*. It is therefore sensible to initiate chemotherapy as soon after surgery as possible. Fears of poor wound healing have been exaggerated in the past; chemotherapy can safely be given as soon as primary wound healing is confirmed, eg one week after laparotomy, although sutures, especially tension sutures, may be left in place during the administration of the drugs if gastro-intestinal side effects, particularly vomiting, are expected.

Immunological status

Surgery, radiotherapy and chemotherapy are known to disturb the immune system. There may be some truth in the essentially basic idea that tumours form initially because of a temporary or permanent defect in the immune system, and even though attempts to manipulate the immune system therapeutically have been largely unsuccessful so far; it is known, for example, that patients suffering from acute leukaemia who are immunocompetent at the beginning of chemotherapy, or become immunocompetent during treatment enter remission, while those who remain immunoincompetent do not (Hersh et al. 1971). Disturbance of the immune system by surgery is inevitable, but it has been shown that even intensive chemotherapy, if given intermittently, can be timed to allow the immune system to recover to some extent between courses of treatment. Ideally, immune support, by immunostimulant drugs for example, given during prolonged and intensive chemotherapy might allow greater and more permanent tumour destruction without detriment to the patient as a whole.

Blood supply

Because cytotoxic drugs reach their target by the blood stream, anything which reduces a tumour's blood supply may compromise the delivery of an effective dose of cytotoxic agents. Furthermore, the reduced blood supply to the tumour promotes hypoxia, and subsequent resistance to therapy. It is thought that chemo-therapy for cancer of the cervix may be compromised by the development of fibrosis and reduction in blood supply in and around the tumour, with consequent hypoxia, induced by radiotherapy. If this is so, chemotherapy for this condition may give better results if given before or during irradiation rather than after.

Radiation sensitisers and protectors

Although not usually regarded as chemotherapy, the use of drugs to enhance or protect against the effects of radiotherapy should be understood; there may one day be applications of a similar nature in chemotherapy. This understanding illustrates the scope available for more widespread integration of anticancer modalities—surgery, radiotherapy, chemotherapy, hormone therapy, immuno-therapy and the enhancement of effect which may be obtained. Drugs which are shown to increase antitumour radiation damage may, in some cases, also promote similar effects when used with standard chemotherapeutic agents.

Read (1952) showed that the radiosensitivity of a cell (in this case a broad bean root cell) is directly related to the availability of oxygen at the time of irradiation rather than to its metabolic state. Gray et al. (1953) indicated the potential therapeutic advantages of this; later it became known that hypoxic cells were relatively resistant to radiation attack (Powers and Tolmach 1963).

Hyperbaric oxygen has been used to combat tumour cell hypoxia during therapy, but the problems encountered have been considerable and the results not especially encouraging. There has also been a search for other electron-attracting compounds which, like oxygen, can sensitise cells by oxidising the free radicals in DNA. Since 1970 two groups of substances appeared to function thus—the 5 nitroimidazoles and the 2 nitroimidazoles, the latter group being ten times more potent than the former. Thus misonidazole and desmethylmisonidazole oxidise neutral radicals in tumour DNA, and the administration of such drugs in tablet form has obvious advantages over irradiation of patients under hyperbaric oxygen. These drugs induce a differential sensitisation because only 0.1% of normal cells are hypoxic, while the proportion in a tumour can be as high as 30%. At the time of writing misonidazole has passed through Phase I and II studies, and Phase III (see Chapter 4) trials are underway in the UK and USA with a view to its use in cases of advanced carcinoma of the cervix.

Radiation protectors

Since the development of nuclear weapons there has been a search for substances to protect troops and civilians against the effects of ionising radiation. Sulphydryl-containing compounds were the first to be found effective (Patt et al. 1949), and later the thiophosphates, of which WR2721 [S-2(3-aminopropyl-amino ethyl phosphorothioic acid hydrate)] seems the most efficient. WR2721 accumulates in normal tissues quicker than in tumours. Radiation protection of normal tissues, eg skin, follows in 30–60 minutes, but tumour concentration takes several hours to build up. Animal studies have shown significant protection in bone marrow, skin, mucous membranes, salivary glands and small gut linings. Phase II studies are in progress.

'Priming'

Additional protection of the small intestine and bone marrow during cytotoxic therapy has been provided by administering a relatively small dose of an alkylating agent; eg cyclophosphamide, which 'primes' the lining cells against high dose cytotoxic therapy given after a specific time interval. This 'John Millar Effect' can be used to protect against the very large doses of ionising irradiation and the massive doses of alkylating agents in use by some centres in London in attempt to thrust highly resistant tumours into regression, and to eradicate resistant tumour stem cells, in patients who have shown good clinical remissions (Millar et al. 1978, Headley and Millar 1978).

The use of these substances has allowed a more flexible approach to the administration of radiotherapy and chemotherapy. They offer an opportunity to improve the cancer treatment we have, rather than to hope (possibly in vain) for the 'magic bullet' total cancer cure drug to come one day. Combinations of cytotoxic chemotherapy, irradiation, radioprotective agents and hypoxic cell sensitisers may be the means of improving therapeutic ratios, and perhaps even the eradication of very advanced tumours which at present usually prove unassailable.

References

Bagley, C. M., Bostick, F. W., De Vita, V. T., Clinical Pharmacology of Cyclophosphamide. *Cancer Res.*, 1973, **33**, 226.

Barker, G. H., Wiltshaw, E., Randomised trial comparing low dose cisplatin and chlorambucil with low dose cisplatin, chlorambucil and doxorubicin in advanced ovarian carcinoma. *Lancet*, 1981, **1**, 747–50.

Connors, T. A., Cox, P. J., Farmer, P. B., Foster, A. B., Jarman, M., Some studies of the active intermediates formed in the microsomal metabolism of cyclophosphamide and iphosphamide. *Biochem. Pharmacol.*, 1974, **23**, 115.

Einhorn, N., Acute leukaemia after chemotherapy (melphalan). *Cancer*, 1978, **41**, 444–7.

Fennelly, J. J., letter, *Cancer Topics*, 3 (10), Jan./Feb. 1982.

Frei, E., Combination cancer therapy. *Cancer Res.*, 1972, **32**,, 2593–607.

Gray, L. H., The concentration of oxygen dissolved in tissues at the time of irradiation as a factor in radiotherapy. *Br. J. Radiol.*, 1953, **26**, 638.

Headley, D., Millar, J. R., McElwain, T., Gordon, M., Acceleration of bone marrow recovery by pretreatment with cyclophosphamide in patients receiving high dose melphalan. *Lancet*, 1978, **2**, 966.

Hersh, E. M., Whitecar, J. P., McCredie, K. B., Bodey, G. P., Freireich, E. J., Chemotherapy, immunoincompetence, immunocompetence and prognosis in acute leukaemia. *New Eng. J. Med.*, 1971, **285**, 1211.

Loo, T. L., Luce, J. K., Sullivan, M. P., Frei, E., Clinical pharmacological observations on 6-mercaptopurine and 6 methyl mercaptopurine ribonucleoside. *Clin. Pharmacol. Ther.*, 1968, **9**, 180.

Millar, J. R., Hudspith, B. N., McElwain, T., Phelps, T. A., Effect of high dose melphalan on marrow and intestinal epithelium in mice pretreated with cyclophosphamide. *Brit. J. Cancer*, 1978, **38**, 137.

Patt, H. M., Tyree, E. B., Straube, R. L., Cysteine protection against X-irradiation. *Science*, 1949, **110**, 213–4.

Pedersen-Bjergaard, J., Nissen, N. I., Sorensen, H. M., Hou-Jensen, K., Larsen, M. S., Ernst, P., Ersbol, J., Knudtzon, S., Rose, C., Acute non-lymphocytic leukaemia in patients with ovarian carcinoma following long-term treatment with treosulphan (=dihydroxybusulfan). *Cancer*, 1980, **45**, 19–29.

Powers, W. E., Tolmach, L. J., A multi-component X-ray survival curve for mouse lymphosarcoma cells irradiated in vivo. *Nature*, 1963, **197**, 710.

Read, J., The effect of ionising radiation on the broad bean root. Part X. *Br. J. Radiol.*, 1952, **25:89**, 154.

Reimer, R. R., Hoover, R., Fraumeni, J. F., Young, R. C., Acute leukaemia after alkylating-agent therapy of ovarian cancer. *New Engl. J. Med.*, 1977, **297**, 177–81.

Chapter Four

Evaluation of Cytotoxic Agents, the Disease and the Patient

Evaluation of cytotoxic agents

New cytotoxic drugs are produced by various means: some are produced synthetically, based upon known anti-tumour formulae; others are natural products from plants, e.g. the vinca alkaloids, or from microorganisms. A few are found by chance, eg cisplatin. Each agent is put through a screening process. They are first tested against a range of experimental animal tumours, eg Lewis lung carcinoma, Walker 256 carcino-sarcoma, L1210 leukaemia; having shown some antitumour activity the drugs are then given preclinical tests proceeding onto *phased* clinical trials. Successful drugs might then reach the market. Even if the cure for all cancer was in the laboratory today it would probably take a decade before it was in widespread use. Needless to say, the costs of research and development of such drugs are colossal and this may be reflected in their eventual retail price.

During 1973, a busy drug screening year, the National Cancer Institute in the USA checked through 51,334 agents, out of which only 13 were selected for clinical trials (Schepartz 1976).

Phase I

This includes trials of active drugs against small animal tumours, eg xenografts in immune depressed mice. They will then go on to patients with very advanced cancer of various types in order to assess toxicity, types and severity, and mode of administration.

Phase II

Trials performed on groups of patients with the same tumour—usually advanced or metastatic—so that response rates may be observed after relatively short time scales. Side effects and toxicity may also be assessed, incorporating phase I trial data.

Phase III

Trials expanding on the phase II results, varying doses, schedules, routes and times of administration.

Staging, grading, and assessment

Staging

Cancer should be thought of in dynamic terms: growing, shrinking and only occasionally static. When cancer is diagnosed every effort should be made to evaluate its size and extent, and every gynaecological malignancy should then be allotted to a FIGO (International Federation of Gynaecologists and Obstetricians) stage. It is only by precise staging, using this internationally agreed system, that results of treatment can be compared between centres, both nationally and internationally. Every hospital must constantly compare its results with others to ensure the treatment it is offering to its cancer patients compares favourably, and that patients are not disadvantaged by attending units with poor results.

If individual centres do not frequently record and review the performance of their patients there is always a danger, particularly in the management of gynaecological malignancy, that the unit will assume its patients are performing better than they really are. There is obviously a tendency to remember the cures seen regularly in outpatient clinics, and forget the failures. Poor results, shown by statistical analysis of patient survival for each treatment modality, often galvanise units into dissatisfaction with so-called 'standard treatments' and promote a desire to improve treatment. No unit in the world has room for complacency in its management of these cancers. Complacency begins when results are assumed rather than checked.

Progression, regression, and recurrence

Once a tumour has been diagnosed and every effort has been made to allot it to a correct stage, that staging cannot be altered. A woman with a malignant pleural effusion and secondary lung deposits has stage IV ovarian carcinoma. If during treatment the extraperitoneal deposits regress and disappear, she does not then have stage III disease; she has stage IV disease with evidence of tumour regression. If having had complete remission from stage I disease for two years, a malignant pleural effusion occurs, then that is not a new stage IV, this must still be regarded as stage I disease but with a late recurrence at a different site.

Since the prognosis of many cancers usually rests with the time, along the path of a tumour's life scale, that the diagnosis was made, the stage of the tumour is similarly related. Staging dictates treatment and indeed prognosis. The necessity of accurate staging cannot be overemphasised. Whereas carcinoma of the cervix is frequently staged carefully, with examination under anaesthetic, cystoscopy, sigmoidoscopy, careful biopsy of tumour and nodes, lymphangiography, excretion urography, liver, bone, brain and lung isotope scanning etc., other tumours, especially ovarian carcinoma and, to some extent, endometrial carcinoma, have frequently been understaged by inadequate assessment, particularly at laparotomy. Such inaccuracy invalidates the assessment of any treatment regimen.

Having recorded accurately and thoroughly the site(s) of initial disease and the extent to which the tumour has been resected by initial surgery, the clinician should have a complete map of the patient's tumour sites and knowledge of tumour dimensions, before commencing further therapy. It is an essential feature of any anticancer chemotherapy that response to treatment is confirmed as early as possible and that if the response is not maintained the drugs are changed, or discontinued. It is unpleasant enough for the patient to receive toxic drugs which are helping to combat her cancer. To give drugs which cannot be seen to be of value to that individual causes needless suffering, and wastes precious time and drugs. Often, different and possibly effective treatment cannot be given immediately but must be delayed a month or even longer until the bone marrow, immune system etc. has recovered sufficiently from the ineffective drugs. Even if no other effective therapy is available, treatment with ineffective cytotoxics should be stopped. It is of no reassurance to a patient to receive repeated courses of a drug which is clearly not proving effective. Many doctors perpetuate ineffective treatment despite disease which is seen to be progressing by the patient, her relatives and by her nurses, on the grounds that they will be reassured by the offer of treatment, however useless. Such doctors, however well intentioned, will eventually be regarded as fools whether they realise it or not.

In the chemotherapy of non-solid tumours such as leukaemia, it is relatively easy to measure and plot response in terms of blood cell numbers. In gynaecological malignancy, responses could until recently be confirmed only in terms of tumour mass reduction, and the disappearance of malignant effusions. However, 'tumour markers' also offer a means of surveillance of some tumours and one day may be applicable to all tumours (see Chapter 5).

Assessment of tumour response to therapy

The following classification is commonly used. However, variations are sometimes introduced so treatment reports should be carefully checked to ensure that the nomenclature used is understood completely.

Complete response (CR) is the complete resolution of all known tumour deposits and malignant effusions.

Partial response is a 50% or more reduction in tumour size, measured as the product of the two maximal perpendicular diameters of the major indicator lesion; no new deposits; complete disappearance of ascites or malignant pleural effusions.

Stasis: no change in size of a major indicator lesion.

Progression: enlargement of lesions and/or the appearance of new ones.

It is essential to ensure that 'stasis' is not, as is often the case, applied to patients with progressive disease which for various reasons has not been detected.

Patient performance status: the Karnofsky score

Initially this was graded by a system introduced by Karnofsky and Burchenal (1949) using 100% as fit and healthy, descending by 10% gradations to 50%, ie requiring considerable assistance and frequent care, down to 10%, ie moribund.

A modern and straightforward grading of patient status has been recommended by the International Union Against Cancer (1977), as follows:

Grade 0 = normal activity, no analgesia
     1 = slight activity restriction, able to carry out light work
     2 = activity restricted but <50% time in bed, unable to work
     3 = severely restricted activity >50% time in bed
     4 = completely disabled

Following up solid tumours

It cannot be too strongly emphasised that no meaningful follow-up of patients can take place, either during or after chemotherapy, unless the exact site and extent of disease at the beginning of therapy is known and recorded. This requires careful staging at diagnosis and, if chemotherapy is commenced sometime after initial staging, any residual or recurrent disease must be measured and recorded.

It is inappropriate to go through every diagnostic procedure required for each stage of each cancer here, but a few examples may illustrate the importance of correct follow-up.

If a patient with recurrent carcinoma of the cervix is about to commence a regimen of chemotherapy and complains of low back pain, spinal secondaries should be suspected. X-rays, isotopic bone scans, and serum hydroxyproline (a breakdown product of damaged collagen from the bone matrix) levels may confirm the presence of such deposits. Their size should be measured and recorded. After a course or two of chemotherapy they should be remeasured. Has a response been clearly demonstrated? Has the pain diminished? Have the secondaries disappeared while a vaginal recurrence has enlarged (a differential response)? Has the primary and all known secondaries disappeared (a complete response)? Indeed, has sufficient time elapsed for the chemotherapy to show some effect?—These are the questions the clinician should be asking before the administration of further chemotherapy.

Facilities for quantifying solid tumours—ultrasound scanning, computerised axial tomography, nuclear magnetic resonance, lymphangiography, isotope scanning etc.—may not be available in every centre, and transfer temporarily, or permanently, to a well equipped specialist centre is strongly recommended. However, initial assessment of disease in the abdomen and pelvis is possible by meticulous search at laparotomy for the site and size of all tumour deposits; subsequent assessments might be made, using interval laparotomy or laparoscopy. The boundaries of inoperable tumours may be located on X-rays by the application of small marker clips at laparotomy.

The use of an operation check-list can be very valuable even for the most experienced surgeon, and has two functions: it facilitates the accurate recording in theatre of known tumour masses; and it reminds the surgeon to check each and

Name .... Number .... Date	Good view	Tumour present	Maximum size of residual tumour	Biopsy taken	Tumour excised	Tissue for xenograft
Ascitic Washings						
Parietal Peritoneum						
Omentum						
Uterus						
Ovaries R.						
L.						
Bladder						
Pelvic peritoneum						
Bowel a) small						
b) mesentery						
c) colon						
d) sigmoid c.						
e) mesocolon						
Nodes: Para-aortic						
Pelvic						
Liver: Surface						
Parenchyma						
Diaphragm R.						
L.						
Other (specify)						

Procedure (e.g. BSO & Hys. & omentectomy)

Comment (please compare appearances with previous operation if possible)

Code: + = tumour   − = clear   o = not done
$\sqrt{}$ = good view or biopsy taken or tumour excised.

Fig. 4.1   Check list for laparotomy or laparoscopy

every site for potential tumour deposits. Figure 4.1 is an example of a check-list Dr Eve Wiltshaw and the author prepared at the Royal Marsden Hospital, London, for use during laparotomy and laparoscopy of patients with ovarian carcinoma:

Because a complete assessment of the patient was made at the beginning of therapy, careful follow-up is possible. Each indicator lesion (and tumour marker, if available) should be checked at frequent intervals. It is often difficult to extract this information from a thick mass of hospital notes and investigations. Dr Eve Wiltshaw and Dr Robert Buckman, at the Royal Marsden Hospital in London,

DATA BASE for: Ca OVARY	NAME:	HOSP No:

DATE OF LAPAROTOMY: 11/3/82 HOSPITAL: St Faiths DATE OF DIAGNOSIS: 11/3/82 DATE OF STUDY ENTRY: 17/3/82

REFERRING HOSP/CONSULT.: Mr Careful	PATH. Nos. (RMH)

	HISTOLOGY: Poorly diff. cyst ad serous

OPERATION PERFORMED: TAH, BSO, OMENTECTOMY

no residual macroscopic tumour left	F.I.G.O. STAGE: III	(AMENDED STAGE IV)

OPERATIVE FINDINGS:	PELVIS Bilat. 12cm diam. ovarian tumours	ASCITES 5 litres
	ABDOMEN ×2 1cm nodules DIAPHRAGM × 3 1cm nodules	BOWEL × 1 2cm nodules
	OMENTUM studded LYMPH NODES nad	LIVER nad

PREVIOUS TREATMENT: Appendicectomy

OBLIGATORY INVESTIGATIONS: MARK ONLY + (FOR ABNORMAL) OR − (FOR NORMAL)

1 Hb + WBC − Plates −	6 PELVIC U/SOUND −	11 Liver isotope scan +
2 U + E − CREAT − LFTS +	7 LIVER U/SOUND +	12
3 CXR −	8 ASCITES CYTOLOGY +	13
4 LYMPHOGRAM −	9 FOR FIGO I & II: LAPAROSCOPY	14
5 IVP −	IF LAPAROTOMY 10 IS PLANNED: C.A.T. SCAN liver +	15

HEIGHT: 165cms	WEIGHT: 70kg	SQ. METRES: 1.65	BLOOD GROUP: OPOS

OTHER INVESTIGATIONS:

1 Gamma GT +	5	9
2 Hep. Surface Ag B −	6	10
3 Ultrasound guided	7	11
4 needle liver biopsy +	8	12

OTHER MEDICAL PROBLEMS—ACTIVE & INACTIVE eg DIABETES, TB, PREVIOUS SURGERY:

PREVIOUS GYNAE DISEASE/OPERATION:

DATE OF DEATH: _____ P.M. No... _____
CAUSE OF DEATH: _____
P.M. FINDINGS _____

Fig. 4.2 Illustration of Data Extraction and Assessment Flow Sheet

You must make an entry on this flow sheet _every time_ *the patient is seen *a course of treatment is given or *any significant event occurs e.g. transfusion record _all_ objective problems e.g. lab results. Girth, liver size &c in figures, record all _subjective_ problems e.g. pain, lymph node size &c in this notation only: ↑ increased ↓ decreased ▨ absent + present = same ± equivocal O not done ↓↑ some parts better, some parts worse

DIAGNOSIS: Ca Ovary Stage IV **SHEET NUMBER** No.: **NAME** _____ **DoB:** __/__/__

DATE	PROBLEM (BLOCK CAPITALS)	ASCITES	LFTS—ALK. PHOS.	GAMMA G.T.	NODULE LIVER ULTRASOUND	NODULE LIVER SCINTISCAN	UREA	MARKER—CEA	HAEMOGLOBIN	TOTAL WBC	PLATELETS	TREATMENT	COURSE NUMBER	INTENDED FREQUENCY—IN WEEKS	
17 3 82	+	↑	↑	+ (2×1)	+		3	↑	8.0	4.0	300	"ZAP"	1	3	TRANSFUSED 3 BLOOD
07 4 82	+	↑	▨	▨	▨		2	▨	11.5	3.8	280	"ZAP"	2	3	NAUSEA Rx MAXOLON
28 4 82	O	↑	↑	+ (1×1)	▨		3	↑	11.0	3.7	200	"ZAP" + "ZIP"	1	4	DIFFERENTIAL RESPONSE . ADD "ZIP"
26 5 82		↓	↓	+ (1×1)			4	↓	9.8	3.2	180	"ZAP" + "ZIP"	2	4	GOOD RESPONSE
23 6 82		↓	▨	O	O		7	↓	7.9	2.9	160	"ZAP" + "ZIP"	3	4	TRANSFUSED 4 BLOOD 4 PLATELETS
21 7 82	NORM	NORM	▨	▨			11	O	12.3	2.8	250	"ZAP" + "ZIP"	4	4	(ON HOLIDAY TO GREECE)
18 8 82	NORM	NORM	O	O			12	▨	11.9	3.0	260	"ZAP" + "ZIP"	5	4	C.R. 1/12
31 8 82	SECOND LOOK LAPAROTOMY—CR CONFIRMED														
15 9 82	NORM	NORM	O	O			12	O	10.9	2.8	210	"ZAP" + "ZIP"	6	4	C.R. 2/12
13 10 82	NORM	▨	▨				17	▨	10.2	2.2	200	"ZAP" + "ZIP"	7	4	C.R. 3/12
10 11 82	NORM	NORM	O	▨			20	O	10.0	2.0	190	TREATMENT STOPPED			C.R. 4/12
8 12 82	NORM	▨	▨	O			19	O	11.0	2.9	220				C.R. 5/12 (SCOTLAND FOR XMAS)
5 1 83	NORM	▨	O	▨			18	O	10.9	3.0	220				C.R. 6/12
2 2 83	▨	▨	▨				16	O	11.3	3.1	280				C.R. 7/12
2 3 83	NORM	▨	O	▨			16	O	11.5	3.1	300				C.R. 8/12
1 4 83	NORM	▨	▨				15	O	▨	▨	▨				C.R. 9/12

INITIAL STATUS

Fig. 4.3

introduced a 'see at a glance' flow sheet system whereby treatment and results are presented in tabular form. Many units use a similar system to extract relevant information, and it makes monitoring patients much easier. In addition, collation of results from all patients undergoing treatment is relatively simple and encourages more frequent reviews of therapy programmes. It is a soul-destroying experience to sit in front of a huge pile of hospital notes with scattered X-ray reports, blood investigations, ultrasound reports etc. and extract information pertinent to the success or otherwise of a treatment schedule; data extraction systems, either by hand or computer linked, are much quicker. Figure 4.2 is an example of a 'flow sheet'.

House officer assessments on admission can be made simple and accurate by flow sheets, and by the use of admission charts for each kind of malignancy (Figures 4.3 and 4.4). It ensures that the relevant information is elicited so that early signs, of, for example, side effects or toxicity, are not overlooked by a failure

OVARIAN CARCINOMA CHEMOTHERAPY ADMISSION CHART

Name: ....   No: ....   Age: ....

Admitted under the care of Dr   on   /   /   for consideration of
chemotherapy course No:...................

consisting of: ....

Since last admission:

D/Q:

Abdo. pain	Mictn.	Appetite
Cough	B.O.	Wheeze
Chest pain	Sputum	SOB
Ankle swelling	Palptns.	Abdo. swelling
Vaginal bleeding		Rectal bleeding
Sleep	Headache	Faints
Paraesthesiae		Sensation

S/H, F/H:

Allergies: Medications:

O/E: Gen. appearance:

Face: Mouth/Throat: Nodes:
Thyroid: Breasts:
Skin: Anaemia:

CVS: P: B/P: /
      JVP: Oedema: H.S.:

R.S.: ct. mvt: PN: Sounds:
       effusions:

Fig. 4.4

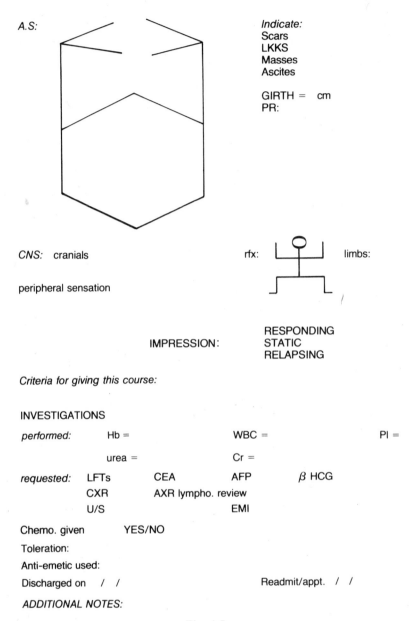

A.S:

Indicate:
Scars
LKKS
Masses
Ascites

GIRTH = cm
PR:

CNS: cranials

peripheral sensation

rfx: limbs:

RESPONDING
IMPRESSION: STATIC
RELAPSING

Criteria for giving this course:

INVESTIGATIONS

performed: Hb =   WBC =   PI =

                urea =   Cr =

requested: LFTs   CEA   AFP   β HCG
               CXR   AXR lympho. review
               U/S   EMI

Chemo. given   YES/NO
Toleration:
Anti-emetic used:
Discharged on   / /   Readmit/appt. / /
ADDITIONAL NOTES:

Fig. 4.5

to question a patient properly. Essential pre-treatment investigations can also be checked at a glance before chemotherapy is administered. Patients with malignancies often have frequent admissions interspersed with outpatient attendances, and thought should be given to the arrangement of their hospital notes; decisions should be written clearly and notes maintained punctually. The patient should be given clear and helpful information about the treatment she is to expect. Figures

4.4 and 4.5 are an example of a formalised admission chart the author prepared for use in the treatment of ovarian carcinoma at the Royal Marsden Hospital.

References

Assessment of response to therapy—advanced breast cancer—a project of the Programme on Clinical Oncology of the International Union Against Cancer. Geneva, Switzerland. Chairman: Haywood, J. L. *Br. J. Cancer*, 1977, **35**, 292–8.

Karnofsky, D. A., Burchenal, J. H., *Evaluation of chemotherapeutic agents*. Ed. C. M. Macleod, Columbia Press, New York, 1949, pp. 191–205.

Schepartz, S. A., Report of the Associate Director, Drug Research and Development. In *The 1976 Report of the Division of Cancer Treatment, National Cancer Institute*, De Vita, V. T., Director, Vol. 1, p. 13, June 1976.

Chapter Five

Tumour Markers

A tumour marker is a substance produced by a cancer which is in some way distinctive. Tumour markers may have a diagnostic as well as follow-up value. Most are, however, of purely research interest. Gilby et al. (1975) have suggested the following criteria of the value of a tumour marker: tumour specificity; concentrations in the blood reflecting extent of disease; produced early in the disease process preferably while disease is subclinical, so that it can be for screening purposes, and easily and cheaply assayed.

In the search for tumour markers four broad areas of interest:

(a) *Oncofetal proteins*, especially carcino-embryonic antigen (CEA) and alpha-fetoprotein (AFP);
(b) *Carcinoplacental proteins*, especially human chorionic gonadotrophin (HCG), the Reagan Isoenzyme (RI), and pregnancy associated β_1 globulin;
(c) *Tumour associated antigens*, especially ovarian cystadenocarcinoma antigen (OCAA);
(d) *Monoclonal antibodies*.

Oncofetal proteins

The explanation that cancer cells put out embryonic proteins is thought to revolve around the loss of regulator gene function associated with rapid cellular growth.

CEA

CEA is a glycoprotein, molecular weight 200 000, initially reported by Gold and Freedman (1965) in patients with carcinoma of the large bowel. It is also produced in low levels in people who do not have cancer. Van Nagell, in Kentucky, estimates that CEA levels greater than 2.5 ng/ml can be found in the blood of 11% of healthy volunteers, 18% of patients with non-malignant gynaecological conditions, 53% of patients with carcinoma of the cervix, 37% of those with endometrial carcinoma and 46% of patients with ovarian carcinoma.

Although there is little diagnostic value in the finding of a raised CEA level, in patients who have a very high level and tumour in the ovaries the possiblity of the tumour being a secondary deposit should be borne in mind and a bowel primary sought.

The value of serial measurement of plasma CEA values in the follow-up of patients with cervical and ovarian tumours is not clear. Some workers, eg Van Nagell et al. (1978), noted that a progressive increase in plasma CEA predicted tumour recurrence in over 80% of patients whose tumour stained immuno-histochemically for CEA. Rising plasma CEA values preceded clinical detection of recurrence by up to six months. Khoo et al. (1979) in Australia found that in 95% of patients with minimal residual ovarian carcinoma after surgical resection, serial CEA levels accurately reflected disease status. However, predictive accuracy fell to 62% in patients with extensive inoperable ovarian cancer. Other workers in London have found any correlation to be of little value (Barker 1980, Stone et al. 1977).

AFP

AFP is a glycoprotein, molecular weight 70 000, discovered by Pederson (1944) and detected in the serum of mice bearing transplantable hepatoma by Abelev (1963), and subsequently in patients with primary liver cancers (Tatarinov 1964). It is also found in patients with tumours containing embryonic tissue, in particular testicular and ovarian germ cell tumours. Its diagnostic value is greatly diminished by its presence in normal maternal serum (Gitlin et al. 1972), although raised where there is fetal abnormality such as neural tube defects. High levels of AFP are found in nearly all cases of ovarian endodermal sinus tumour (Kurman and Norris 1976). Elevated human levels have been found in non-malignant conditions such as hepatitis, cirrhosis of the liver, and obstructive jaundice. There is usually a good correlation between AFP levels and disease status in the follow-up of patients with endodermal sinus tumours. It must be remembered that in mixed germ cell cancers the decline in serum AFP (see Figure 5.1) may indicate only selective response of the endodermal sinus elements to therapy despite the persistence of other extra-embryonal tissue (see Chapter 13).

Carcinoplacental proteins

HCG

HCG is a glycoprotein composed of two polypeptide chains, alpha and beta. The alpha chain is also common to other polypeptides including luteinising hormone. However, their beta subunits are different. Vaitukaitis et al. (1972) developed a specific radio-immunoassay for the beta subunit of HCG.

HCG is quantitatively increased in trophoblastic tumours, and values in excess of 300 000 mIU/ml are indicative of trophoblastic disease (Dawood et al. 1977). So predictable is the release of this marker into the serum that failure to return to normal by eight weeks following evacuation of trophoblastic tissue from the uterus indicates the need for chemotherapy. The response to the chemotherapy is mirrored by the subsequent rise or fall in HCG levels. Thus HCG fulfils almost all of the criteria for a valuable tumour marker—would that each tumour had a similar indicator of therapeutic success or failure! (See Chapter 14.)

RI

RI, the Reagan Isoenzyme, is a placental type of alkaline phosphatase, molecular weight 120 000 (Stolbach et al. 1969). Various authors indicate its incidence in

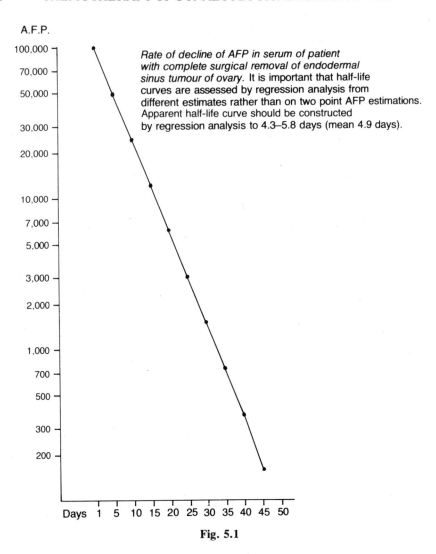

A.F.P.

Rate of decline of AFP in serum of patient with complete surgical removal of endodermal sinus tumour of ovary. It is important that half-life curves are assessed by regression analysis from different estimates rather than on two point AFP estimations. Apparent half-life curve should be constructed by regression analysis to 4.3–5.8 days (mean 4.9 days).

Fig. 5.1

25% of patients with cervical carcinoma, 32% with ovarian carcinoma and 11% with endometrial carcinoma. Although its concentration is directly proportional to extent of disease, the enzyme also appears in the bloodstream of patients suffering from a variety of non-malignant inflammatory conditions such as hepatitis, colitis, and this severely limits its diagnostic value. Serial estimations have, however, been used to follow response to therapy.

Pregnancy associated (β_1) globulin

This has recently been shown to correlate well with the extent of trophoblastic disease and may well be used as a tumour marker in addition to HCG (Atkinson 1981, Bagshawe et al. 1978).

Tumour associated antigens

Although a number of tumour associated antigens have been discovered since 1970, many of which are allegedly diagnostic of ovarian carcinoma, only three are detectable by radio-immunoassay.

Ovarian cystadenocarcinoma antigen (OCAA) documented by Bhattacharya and Barlow (1972 & 1978) is a mucoprotein of large molecular weight. It was present in 60% of patients with early stage disease and in 80% with advanced disease. Its concentration in the blood correlates with the volume and extent of disease, and normal levels are usually achieved within three weeks of total excision. It may prove of value in monitoring patients for early signs of relapse from remission following chemotherapy.

Ovarian cancer antigen (OCA) described by Knauf and Urbach (1974 & 1978) is a glycoprotein of high molecular weight. Knauf and Urbach found significantly raised levels of OCA in the blood of over 60% of patients, and in only 14% of those with benign gynaecological conditions. They also claim a satisfactory relationship with tumour burden.

Cervical squamous cell carcinoma antigen (TA-4) initially reported by Kato et al. (1979) has a molecular weight of 48 000. TA-4 has been detected in normal cervical tissue but it is not found in the blood of patients who do not have cervical cancer. Series have shown raised serum levels in about half of patients with cervical cancer, with successively falling levels following clinical regression.

Monoclonal antibodies

In 1975 Kohler and Milstein first reported the immortalisation of specific-antibody forming cells by somatic cell hybridisation in mice. Olsson and Kaplan (1980) have joined a human myeloma cell to a human spleen cell to produce human monoclonal antibody. This may, in the future, assist with the detection and measurement of tumour associated antigens. Several workers have already produced mouse antibodies against some human tumours. Highly tumour specific antibodies may eventually be labelled with isotope to allow accurate localisation of tumour, including, perhaps, micrometastases. It is possible that eventually cytotoxic drugs or toxins might then be attached (Blythman et al. 1981) to the tumour specific antibody which would be exclusively taken up by the tumour, effecting lethal damage without destroying normal tissue—the so-called 'letter bomb' chemotherapy. The future prospects of monoclonal antibodies in gynaecological oncology may well be of great benefit and are worthy of attention.

References

Abelev, G. I., Study of the antigenic structure of tumors. *Acta Intern. Cancer*, 1963, **19**, 80–92.

Atkinson, R. J., Tumour markers in the detection of gynaecological cancer. *Brit. J. Hosp. Med.*, October 1981, 381–6.

Bagshawe, K. D., Lequin, R. M., Sizaret, P. H., Tatarinov, Y. S., Pregnancy β_1 globulin and chorionic gonadotrophin in the serum of patients with trophoblastic and nontrophoblastic tumours. *Europ. J. Cancer*, 1978, **14**, 1331.

Barker, G. H., in *Controversies in gynaecological oncology*. Proceedings, Royal College of Obstetricians and Gynaecologists, 22nd February, 1980.

Bhattacharya, M., Barlow, J. J., Ovarian tumour antigens. *Cancer*, 1978, **42**, 1616–20.

Beler, G. I., Study of the antigenic structure of tumours. *Acta. Intern. Cancer*, 1963, **19**, 80–92.

Blythman, H. E., Casellas, P., Gros, O., Gros, P., Jansen, F. K., Paolucci, F., Pau, B., Vidal, H., Immunotoxins: hybrid molecules of monoclonal antibodies and a toxin subunit specifically to kill tumour cells. *Nature*, 1981, **290**, 145–6.

Dawood, M. Y., Saxena, B. B., Landesman, R., Human chorionic gonadotrophin and its subunits in hydatidiform mole and choriocarcinoma. *Obstet. Gynecol.*, 1977, **50**, 172–81.

Gilby, E. D., Rees, L. H., Bondy, P. K., in: *Biological characterisation of human tumours*. Ed. Malton C., Davis, W., Elsevier, New York, 1975, p. 132.

Gitlin, D., Perricelli, A., Gitlin, G. M., Synthesis of alpha fetoprotein by liver, yolk sac and gastrointestinal tract of the human conceptus. *Cancer Res.*, 1972, **32**, 979–82.

Gold, P., Freedman, S. O., Demonstration of tumour specific antigens in human colonic carcinoma by immunological tolerance and absorption techniques. *J. Exp. Med.*, 1965, **121**, 439–62.

Kato, H., Miyaghi, F., Marioka, H., Fujino, T., Torigae, T., Tumour antigen of human cervical squamous cell carcinoma. Correlation of circulating levels with disease progress. *Cancer*, 1979, **43**, 585–90.

Khoo, S. K., Whitaker, S. V., Jones, I. S. C., Mackay, E. V., Predictive value of serial CEA levels in the long term follow up of ovarian cancer. *Cancer*, 1979, **43**, 2471–8.

Knauf, S., Urbach, G. I., The development of a double antibody radio-immunoassay for detecting ovarian tumour associated antigen fraction OCA in Plasma. *Am. J. Obstet. Gynecol.*, 1978, **131**, 780–6.

Knauf, S., Urbach, G. I., Ovarian tumour specific antigens. *Am. J. Obstet. Gynecol.*, 1974, **119**, 966–70.

Kohler, G., Milstein, C., Continuous cultures of fused cells secreting antibody of predefined specificity. *Nature*, 1975, **256**, 495.

Kurman, R. J., Norris, H. J., Endodermal sinus tumour of ovary. *Cancer*, 1976, **38**, 2404–19.

Olsson, L., Kaplan, H., Human-human hybridomas producing monoclonal antibodies of predefined antigenic specificity. *Proceedings of the Natl. Academy of Sciences of the USA*, 1980, **77** (9), 5429.

Pedersen, K. O., Fetuin, new globulin isolated from serum. *Nature*, 1944, **154**, 575.

Stolbach, L. L., Krant, M. J., Fishman, W. H., Ectopic production of an alkaline phosphatase iso-enzyme in patients with cancer. *N. Engl. J. Med.*, 1969, **281**, 757–62.

Stone, M., Bagshawe, K. D., Kardana, A., Searle, F., Dent, J., Beta human chorionic gonadotrophin and carcinoembryonic antigen in the management of ovarian carcinoma. *Br. J. Obstet. Gynae.*, 1977, **84**, 375–9.

Tatarinov, J. S., Presence of embryonal α globulin in the serum of a patient with primary hepatocellular carcinoma. *Vop. Med. Khim*, 1964, **1**, 90–1.

Vaitukaitis, J. L., Braunstein, G. P., Ross, G. T., A radio-immunoassay which specifically measures human chorionic gonadotrophin in the presence of luteinising hormone. *Am. J. Obstet. Gynecol.*, 1972, **113**, 751–6.

Van Nagell, J. R., Donaldson, E. S., Wood, E. C., Goldenberg, D. M., The clinical significance of carcino-embryonic antigen in the plasma and tumours of patients with gynaecologic malignancies. *Cancer*, 1978, **42**, 1527–32.

Chapter Six

Treatment Efficacy, Analysis and Trials

Presentation of results

The effectiveness of chemotherapies can be compared at any time during or after a treatment programme. All clinicians should be able to interpret the results and realise their implications. The method of presenting such results largely depends on the nature of the cancer. In a cancer which is relatively difficult to treat chemotherapeutically, eg advanced malignancies of the head and neck, results may be presented as response rates over periods as short as two or three months. In more successfully treated tumours, results can be expressed in years of survival after diagnosis. This may be qualified further by separating disease-free survival from crude survival rates; a patient with a tumour may remain alive for some considerable time.

Response rates are frequently expressed as median response times, eg median CR 18 months, range 6 to 28 months.

Survival can be shown using a survival curve plotted over a time interval (which some authors extrapolate to give a projected or 'guessed' survival rate for the future beyond the length of the current trial) or as a survival rate after a fixed time interval, eg 2, 5 or 10 years.

Life table method

In many trials of chemotherapeutic agents for gynaecological malignancies patients cannot all start at the beginning of the trial period. Patients usually enter such trials at different times and, indeed, may leave, eg die, or change to different therapy, before the end of it. Patients who are entered after the start of the trial will not have been followed up for as long as patients entered earlier. Therefore to compare, say, the efficacy of two chemotherapy treatments eg 'ZAP' and 'FLOP' in a tumour of a certain stage, over a trial period of, say, three years, crude survival times may be unhelpful. Instead, a life table should be constructed, and a survival curve plotted from it. The trial period is divided into suitable intervals, eg 6 months. The trial report can be made when the drugs have been given to a certain number of patients, or after a certain minimum length of follow up. Figure 6.1 shows the survival curve after 50 patients have been treated with each drug, with a minimum follow up of 6 months. At any time interval after entry into the trial the probability of death (and conversely survival) can be determined for all those patients who have survived the preceding interval. As the trial proceeds and more deaths occur, say from late relapses, the cumulative probability of surviving to the end, say, of the third year may become quite low.

Often the actual number of patients entering each interval (ie survivors) is included in brackets. One can see that treatment with 'ZAP' seems better than with 'FLOP', and that the prognosis seems good for patients who survive the first year. However, the prediction may not be correct and later relapses may occur,

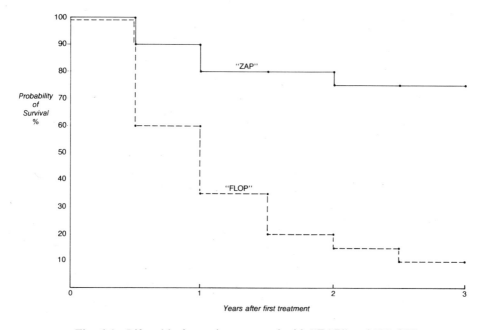

Fig. 6.1   Life table for patients treated with "ZAP" and "FLOP"

and with follow up, as compared to predictions, both survival curves may converge later, say at the 5 to 6 year mark.

The statistical method used in the comparison of survival curves is based on the χ^2 test. The χ^2 statistics for each interval can be accumulated to produce a summary χ^2 statistic for each treatment group (Mantel, 1966) which enables the comparison of survival probability amongst several different treatment groups. It is also possible to adjust differences among subgroups in order to make allowances for prognostic factors such as degrees of differentiation of tumour, age of patient etc.

The design, ethics, conduct and evaluation of such trials have been very fully discussed in a recent Medical Research Council Report and the reader is recommended to study this in full (Peto et al. 1976 & 1977).

References

Mantel, N., Evaluation of survival data and two new rank order statistics arising in its consideration. *Cancer Chemother. Rep.*, 1966, **50**, 163–70.

Peto, R., Pike, M. C., Armitage, P., Breslow, N. E., Cox, D. R., Howard, S. V., Mantel, N., McPherson, K., Peto, J., Smith, P. G., Design and analysis of randomised clinical trials requiring prolonged observation of each patient 1. Introduction and Design 1. Analysis and example. *Brit. J. Cancer*, 1976, **34**, 585–612; *Brit. J. Cancer*, 1977, **35**, 1–39.

Chapter Seven

The Basic Pharmacology of Anti-neoplastic Drugs

Alkylating agents

The essential action of alkylating agents is to form covalent bonds to cell molecules with alkyl groups—especially to the bases in deoxyribonucleic acid (DNA), cross linking the two strands of the double helix. Their effectiveness may be reduced if the alkylated groups are jettisoned by the action of enzymes called the endonucleases.

Half lives of alkylating agents are usually short and this has therapeutic value (see p. 138). Many alkylating agents contain two alkylating groups in each molecule and are thus referred to as bifunctional alkylating agents. Alkylating agents are considered to be cell cycle phase non-specific but they are undoubtedly more toxic to rapidly proliferating cells than to other cells.

There are five major groups of alkylating agents: nitrogen mustards, triazenes, methane sulphonic acid esters, ethylenimines, and nitrosoureas.

Nitrogen mustards

Mechlorethamine (nitrogen mustards, HN₂)

$$H_3C\text{—}N\begin{cases} CH_2\text{—}CH_2\text{—}Cl \\ CH_2\text{—}CH_2\text{—}Cl \end{cases}$$

Mechlorethamine is soluble in water and has a very rapid action. It is usually administered intravenously via a fast running drip. The other alkylating agents are more lipophilic and therefore slower reacting and may be given orally, since absorption and distribution in the body can occur before they react with nucleophile groups. The agent is very vesicant and care should be taken not to cause extravasation or spill onto the skin of either patient or staff. Other side effects are mostly confined to nausea and vomiting; its dose-limiting toxicity is bone marrow depression. It was first used clinically in November 1942 on a patient with lymphosarcoma (Gilman 1963). Its use is now almost exclusively in the treatment of Hodgkin's disease.

Chlorambucil

$$HOOC-(CH_2)_3-\langle\bigcirc\rangle-N\begin{matrix}CH_2-CH_2-Cl\\CH_2-CH_2-Cl\end{matrix}$$

Chlorambucil, synthesised in the early 1950s at the Chester Beatty Research Institute in London by Prof W. C. J. Ross and his colleagues, is a phenylbutyric derivative of nitrogen mustard (Everett et al. 1953). It is administered orally, usually daily. Its myelosuppressive action is usually moderate, gradual and reversible. Prolonged continuous administration, like many other alkylating agents, may be associated with the development of acute myelogenous leukaemia. Intermittent therapy, eg alternate fortnights, reduces this risk considerably. It is well tolerated with only occasional reports of gastrointestinal upset. Chlorambucil is used in the treatment of chronic lymphocytic leukaemia, primary (Waldenstrom's) macroglobulinaemia and ovarian carcinoma.

Cyclophosphamide

$$\begin{matrix}H&H&H\\ &C-N&\\H&&\\ &C&O=P-N\quad\begin{matrix}CH_2-CH_2-Cl\\CH_2-CH_2-Cl\end{matrix}\\H&C-O&\\ &H&H\end{matrix}$$

Cyclophosphamide was developed in Europe during the search for, and development of, a nitrogen mustard which was more selective for neoplastic tissues (Arnold and Bourseaux 1958). It can be administered intravenously or orally (70–80% absorbed). It is activated by enzymes in the liver and plasma, which split the cyclic groups at the phosphorus-nitrogen bond to produce several active metabolites (Connors et al. 1974). It has a plasma half life of 6.5 hours in patients who have not received the drug before (Bagley et al. 1973). Cyclophosphamide is excreted mostly in the faeces but some 17% is excreted in the urine, frequently producing a form of recognisable cystitis which can be troublesome long after the drug has been discontinued. A high fluid throughput is therefore recommended during administration to reduce the intravesical concentration—however, the effect is not just local and epithelial linings throughout the body are to some extent affected. High dose intravenous therapy is usually associated with nausea, some vomiting and alopecia. These side effects are less marked with low dose oral therapy. Cyclophosphamide can cause amenorrhoea, ovarian and testicular destruction in standard doses (Barker 1982). Its immunosuppressive ability, especially its lowering of circulating B and T lymphocytes, has been used in such non-malignant conditions as rheumatoid arthritis and dermatomyositis. It is a popular drug for use in ovarian cancer either as a single agent or in combination with other cytotoxic drugs.

Iphosphamide (Ifosfamide)

Iphosphamide is an isomer of cyclophosphamide which has produced responses in tumours of the lung, ovary, breast, gut, kidney, endometrium and bone (Brock and Scheef 1972). Its side effects and toxicity are similar to cyclophosphamide except that its most serious and dose limiting toxicity is haemorrhagic cystitis which occurs in 40–50% of patients (Van Dyk et al. 1972). However, attempts have been made to reduce this cystitis by concurrent administration of ascorbic acid and other reducing agents, forced diuresis and dose fractionisation (Rodriguez et al. 1976).

Melphalan

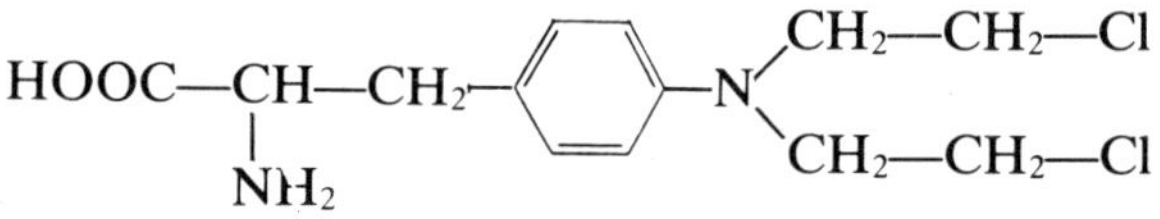

$$HOOC-CH-CH_2-\bigcirc-N\begin{array}{c}CH_2-CH_2-Cl\\CH_2-CH_2-Cl\end{array}$$
$$\underset{NH_2}{\quad}$$

L-phenylalanine mustard, or L-PAM, was synthesised in the early 1950s (at the Chester Beatty Research Institute in London) with the largely unfulfilled hope of using it effectively against malignant melanoma, since phenylalanine is a precursor of melanin (Bergel and Stock 1953). However, interest in its other cytotoxic properties quickly generated in centres such as the Royal Marsden Hospital in London (Wiltshaw and Galton 1958), Italy, Germany, the USA and Russia (Trusheikina 1956). It is administered orally or intravenously and is well tolerated. Nausea and vomiting are uncommon in small dose regimens and it does not cause significant alopecia. However, it is myelotoxic. Principal uses include the treatment of myelomatosis, although it has had extensive use in the management of breast and ovarian cancers, especially in the USA.

Busulphan

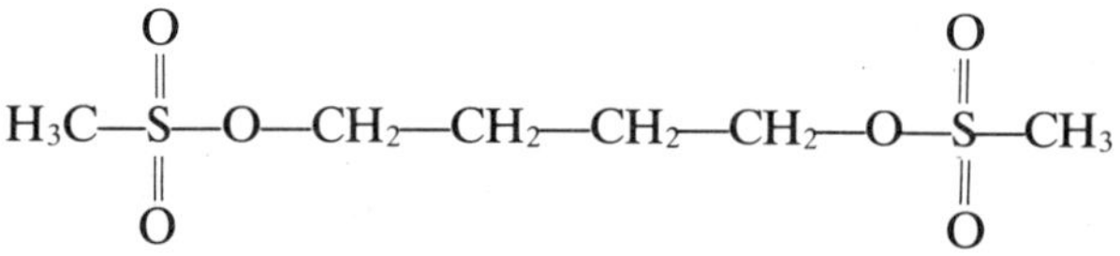

$$H_3C-\overset{O}{\underset{O}{\overset{\|}{\underset{\|}{S}}}}-O-CH_2-CH_2-CH_2-CH_2-O-\overset{O}{\underset{O}{\overset{\|}{\underset{\|}{S}}}}-CH_3$$

Busulphan was one of the most useful of the methane sulphonic acid esters developed at the Chester Beatty Research Institute in London (Haddow and Timmis 1951). Effects may be altered by changes in methylene bridge length ($n = 2$ to 10); the compounds of intermediate length ($n = 4$ or 5) possess the highest therapeutic indices. Its selective action against granulocytes was noted, leading, in 1953, to its successful use against chronic granulocytic leukaemia (Galton 1953).

Treosulphan

Research workers at the Chester Beatty Research Institute in London were looking for more polar analogues of busulphan which might be equally cytotoxic but less myelosuppressive, and as a result, synthesised the 1,6-dimethane-sulphonate of D-mannitol (Haddow et al. 1958). It was found to have a cytotoxic activity pattern different from that of busulphan. Eventually chemists from Leo Laboratories in Copenhagen synthesised the 1,4-dimethane sulphonate of L-threitol, a similar analogue, and it was this that was selected for further investigation in the USA. It was only later discovered that this compound, treosulphan, was converted in vivo to L-diepoxybutane which was the active drug and which has been known to be mutagenic since the 19th century. The conversion requires an alkaline pH and therefore treosulphan remains inactive in the stomach until absorption into the blood-stream (Burnett 1982).

$$CH_3O_2SO—CH_2—CH—CH—CH_2OSO_2CH_3$$
$$\overset{|}{OH} \quad \overset{|}{OH}$$

treosulphan

Treosulphan is administered orally, usually daily for alternate months in order to allow bone marrow recovery and decrease the risk of leukaemic development. Its activity is due to the formation of epoxide compounds in vivo. It is well tolerated although, rarely, some patients experience nausea, mild allergic reactions, and stomatitis if the capsules are chewed rather than swallowed as recommended. Between a quarter and one half of patients treated experience a generalised pigmentation which is usually not unwelcome. Its main use is in the treatment of ovarian cancer.

Triethylene thiophosphoramide (ThioTEPA)

Because the initial reaction of mechlorethamine in water involves the ionization of chloride and the formation of the ethylene immonium ion, research was directed to finding active ethylenimine derivatives. The anticancer effects in humans of triethylene melamine (TEM) were first described in 1950 (Rhoads et al. 1950, Wright et al. 1950). TEM was initially synthesised by industrial chemists for use in improving the finish of rayon fabrics. Others were introduced later: triethylene phosphoramide (TEPA) and triethylene thiophosphoramide (thioTEPA) (Shay et al. 1953).

$$\begin{array}{c} H_2C—CH_2 \\ \diagdown \quad \diagup \\ CH_2 \quad N \\ \diagdown \quad | \\ \quad N—P{=}S \qquad thioTEPA \\ \diagup \quad | \\ CH_2 \quad N \\ \diagup \quad \diagdown \\ CH_2—CH_2 \end{array}$$

ThioTEPA acts like an alkylating agent, is poorly absorbed through the gut and is given intravenously or topically, as in the bladder, peritoneal or pleural cavities. However, its intraperitoneal or intrapleural action is not sclerosing and there is little advantage, if any, in this route over giving the agent intravenously. It frequently causes bone marrow depression, anorexia, nausea, vomiting, and occasionally local pain at the injection site. It has widespread use in advanced ovarian carcinoma, but it has been largely superseded by more effective agents.

Hexamethylmelamine

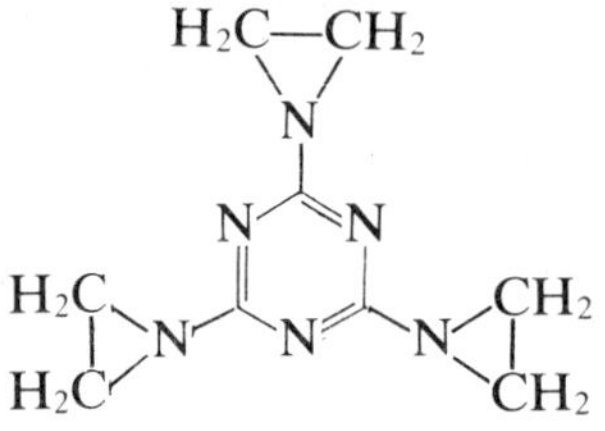

triethylenemelamine (TEM) 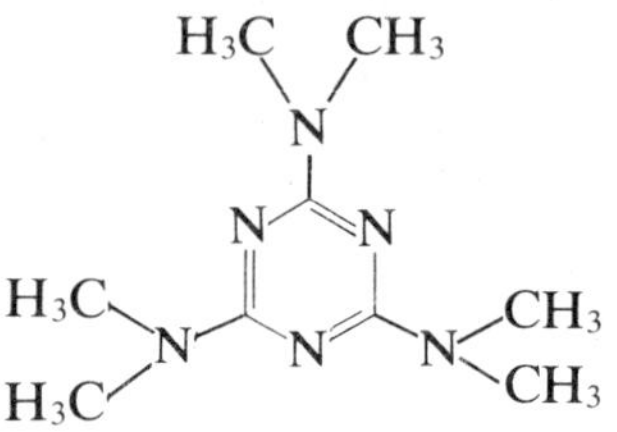   hexamethylmelamine (HMM)

Although similar in structure to that of the alkylating agent triethylenemelamine (TEM), hexamethylmelamine (HMM), synthesised at the Chester Beatty Research Institute, in London, does not appear to act in the same way, and has been shown to inhibit the incorporation of precursors into DNA and RNA (Heere and Donnelly 1971).

It is readily absorbed orally, metabolised and excreted in the urine, with a plasma half life of approximately 13 hours (Worzella et al. 1974). Side effects, mostly nausea and vomiting, are common, occasionally in association with abdominal cramps and diarrhoea. It is neurotoxic and may cause parasthesia, hyporeflexia, muscle weakness, and ataxia which are reversible, and, in some cases, reduced by the administration of pyridoxine. Moderate myelosuppression may also occur.

Early trials showed significant activity in cancers of the ovary, cervix and endometrium (Legha et al. 1976).

Pentamethylmelamine is also being investigated. It is more soluble than HMM and was hoped to be less toxic and clinically more effective, but early trials so far have not substantiated those aims.

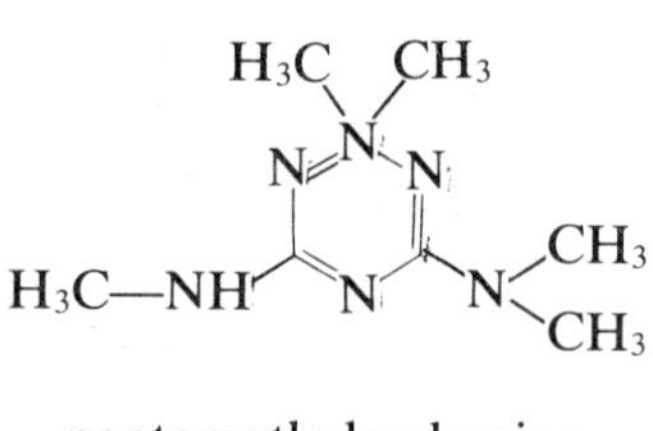

pentamethylmelamine

Nitrosoureas

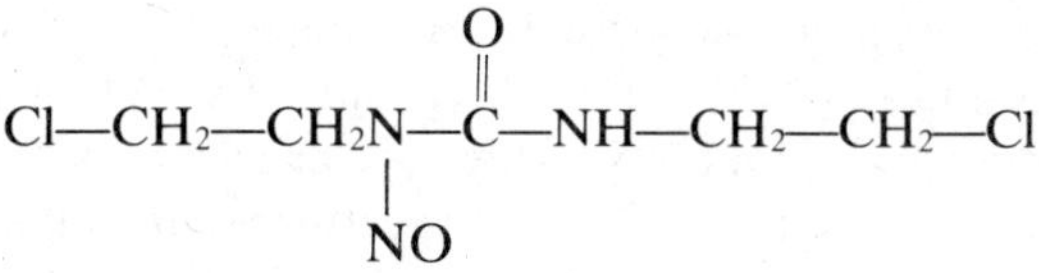

$$\underset{\displaystyle \underset{NO}{|}}{Cl-CH_2-CH_2N}-\overset{\displaystyle \overset{O}{\|}}{C}-NH-CH_2-CH_2-Cl$$

Carmustine (BCNU)

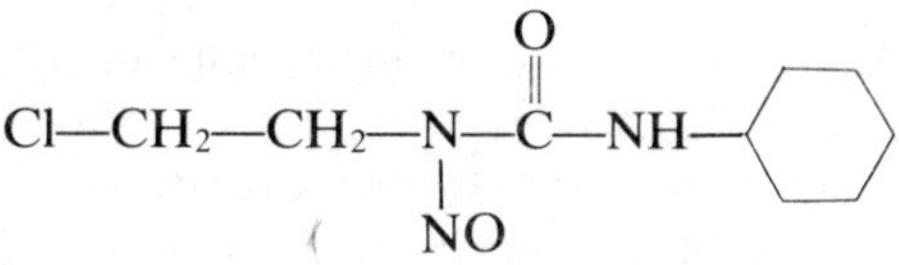

Lomustine (CCNU)

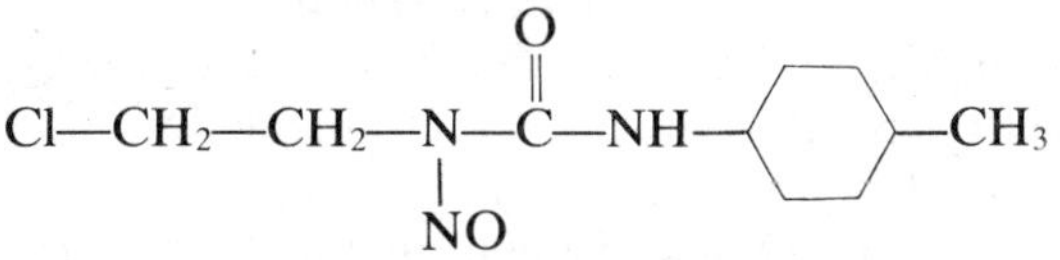

Semustine (methyl CCNU)

Nitrosoureas act similarly to the nitrogen mustards and are both alkylating as well as carbamoylating ie attach an alkyl ($R—CH_2$) or a carbamoyl ($R—N—C=O$) moiety. They are rapidly absorbed from the gastrointestinal tract and, after metabolism, are excreted principally in the urine. In contrast to other alkylating agents they are very lipophilic and therefore can readily cross the blood brain barrier and into the cerebrospinal fluid. Their major toxicity is leukopenia and thrombocytopoenia, which is delayed and cumulative, and side effects include nausea and vomiting. Their main use has been in the treatment of primary and secondary intracerebral tumours, Hodgkin's disease and melanoma (Wasserman et al. 1975).

Cisplatin

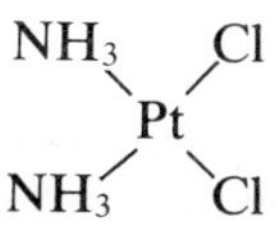

cis-dichlorodiammineplatinum (II)

It was by chance that Rosenberg in the USA (1965), investigating the effects of an electrical field on bacterial growth processes, noted an inhibition of the growth of *Escherichia coli*. Subsequent investigation showed that the inhibition was due to a family of inorganic compounds formed in solution from platinum dissolved from the electrodes. Rosenberg and his colleagues (1969) capitalised on this observation and cisplatin became the first of a generation of platinum-based antitumour agents; other members of the same family of platinum-based drugs are now under investigation (Rosenweig et al. 1977). This chemical was originally synthesised in 1845 and was known as Peyrone's chloride. The exact mode of action is unknown but cisplatin appears to act in all stages of the cell cycle. It inhibits DNA synthesis, possibly by cross linking complementary strands of DNA in the nucleus (Roberts and Pascoe 1972), binding preferentially to guanine and also to adenine and cytosine.

It is administered intravenously in a single bolus or by short infusion and is eliminated via a biphasic plasma clearance pattern with an initial half life of 30 minutes and a secondary half life of 60–70 hours (Barker 1980). Side effects are mainly gastrointestinal: nausea, vomiting and diarrhoea are common, especially when high doses are given. Alopecia is uncommon. Hypersensitivity reactions have also been reported, although cisplatin itself is immunosuppressive (Khan et al. 1975). Myelosuppression is moderate—a normochromic, normocytic anaemia is not uncommon when high doses are used (Barker 1979). Cisplatin may also produce a dose dependent ototoxicity with hearing loss most prominent at high frequencies (over 4000 Hz) (Piel et al. 1974). Prolonged high dose administration may also cause a reversible sensory neuropathy of the fingers and toes (Barker 1979). Heavy metal compounds are well known for their ability to produce renal failure, and, as with cisplatin, produce a renal toxicity, manifested by elevation of the plasma urea and creatinine, which is dose related and cumulative. However, the renal hazards of high dose administration of cisplatin have been overcome by prehydrating the patient with normal saline and the promotion of a post-treatment diuresis with mannitol solutions (Hayes et al. 1977), or by giving doses divided over several days, since low dose administration with adequate fluid replacement does not produce significant nephrotoxicity (Barker and Wiltshaw 1981). Cisplatin has shown considerable activity in advanced ovarian carcinoma and some potential in carcinoma of the cervix. In combination with vinblastine and bleomycin, it produces prolonged, complete remissions in a very large proportion of young men with disseminated testicular tumours. It has also been used in the management of advanced bladder tumours and cancers of the head and neck.

Antimetabolites

Of the three groups of antimetabolites in clinical use, folic acid analogues, antipyrimidines and antipurines, the first is of great importance, not only to those interested in gynaecological malignancies, but to oncologists in all areas of human cancer treatment. The exciting report from the USA that Farber et al. (1948) had produced a marked, but only temporary, remission of acute leukaemia in children with aminopterin was a significant and encouraging step in the development of cancer chemotherapy. Methotrexate (amethopterin), another folic acid antagonist, was later shown to produce long-lasting remissions in choriocarcinoma (Li et al. 1956). Prior to such chemotherapy choriocarcinoma almost invariably caused death within a year of diagnosis. Later workers went on to demonstrate that a single chemotherapeutic agent, without surgery or radiotherapy, could produce cures in even women with very widespread disease, and gives great encouragement to seek similar agents or combinations thereof with comparable performance in other tumours.

Methotrexate

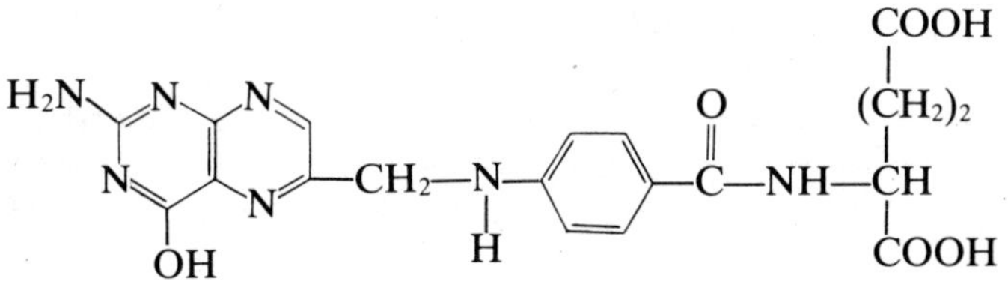

folic acid

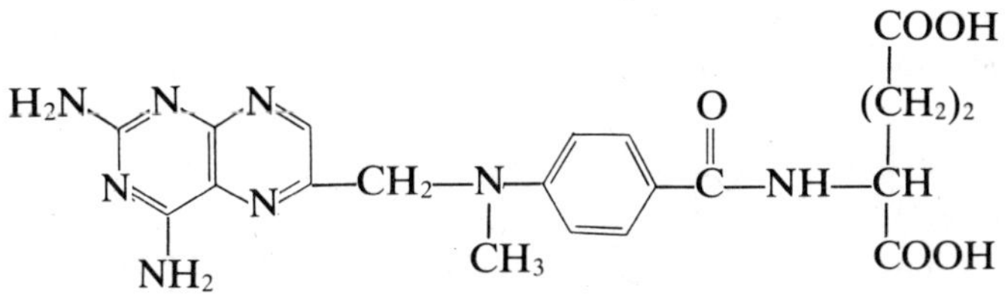

methotrexate

DIHYDROFOLIC ACID

dihydrofolate reductase

NADPH

NADP

TETRAHYDROFOLIC ACID

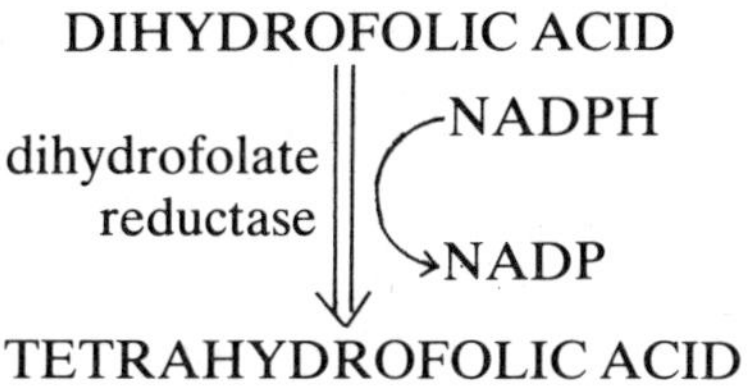

Methotrexate is a powerful competitive inhibitor of dihydrofolate reductase—the enzyme which reduces dihydrofolic acid to tetrahydrofolic acid (in the presence of NADPH) before the latter can accept a one-carbon unit and act as a coenzyme in the synthesis of thymidylate purines, methionine and glycine, necessary for DNA synthesis. Methotrexate is thus an S-phase specific agent.

Methotrexate binds folate reductases from normal and cancer cells with the same affinity. High concentrations of methotrexate can be tolerated providing the duration of exposure is not prolonged (eg 24 hours or less). Folinic acid, a tetrahydrofolate derivative (leucovorin, citrovorum factor), can then be administered in large doses to bypass the methotrexate blockade and restore thymidylate and purine synthesis. This is referred to as 'folinic acid rescue'. High doses may well be required as resistance to methotrexate can result secondary to increased dihydrofolate reductase production and/or decreased cell membrane permeability to methotrexate.

Methotrexate can be administered orally, intravenously, intrathecally (since little of the drug enters the CSF from the blood) and intra-arterially to provide local perfusion. While good levels in the plasma are obtained when low doses are given orally, high doses are best administered directly into the bloodstream.

Between 50% and 90% of the drug (depending upon the dose given) is excreted in the urine within 48 hours, most of it in the first 8 hours. However, the remainder is retained for long periods and gradually excreted in the urine over a matter of weeks or months. Patients with impaired renal function must be treated with caution, therefore. Enzymatic and immuno-assays are available for drug level monitoring.

Methotrexate is usually well tolerated, especially in low doses, but anorexia, nausea and diarrhoea are common. A small proportion of patients may develop a maculo-papular rash on the upper trunk and neck. Alopecia and osteoporosis can also occur.

Intrathecal administration may cause meningism and neurotoxicity.

Methotrexate causes myelosuppression and toxic effects on the endothelium of the oropharynx and lower intestinal tract. Toxic reactions may vary from mild erythema to severe ulceration of the buccal mucosa and oropharynx, and from mild diarrhoea to severe haemorrhagic desquamating enteritis. High dose administration can also cause kidney and liver damage. The effects of folic acid analogues on embryogenesis are discussed in Chapter 8.

In addition to its use in trophoblastic disease and acute lymphocytic leukaemia of children, methotrexate is also of value in the treatment of advanced carcinoma of the cervix and vulva. It has also been used in osteogenic sarcoma, tumours of the head and neck, breast cancer and in the non-malignant diseases of systemic lupus erythematosis, psoriasis, and Wegener's granulomatosis, for its immuno-suppressive activity.

Purine analogues

purine   6-mercaptopurine

Following research in World War II a number of natural purine base analogues have been investigated which were hoped to interfere with the biosynthesis of nucleotides. The most important of these was 6-mercaptopurine, first described by Elion and her colleagues (1952), and its antileukaemic properties in children first described a year later (Burchenal et al. 1953). Its addition to the existing treatment increased the proportion of children surviving longer than one year to over 50%, whereas 90% were previously expected to die within one year.

Although 6-mercaptopurine has not been helpful in the management of solid tumours its imidazoyl derivative, azathiaprine, has been widely used as an immunosuppressant in the prevention of transplanted organ rejection.

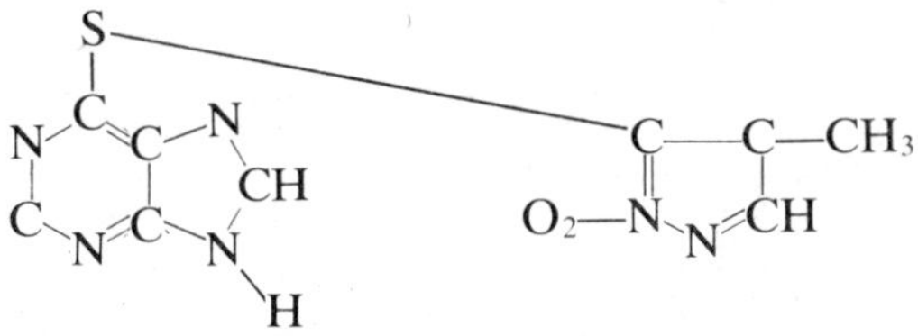

azathiaprine

Pyrimidine analogues

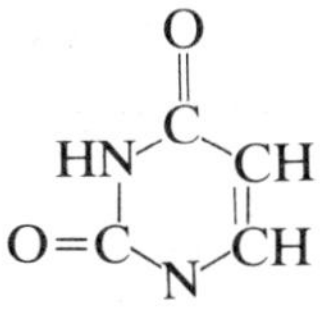

uracil 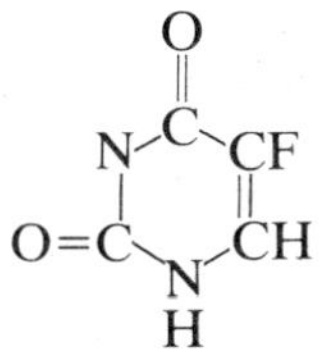   5-fluorouracil

5-fluorouracil was designed systematically by Heidelberger and his coworkers in 1957 (Duschinsky et al. 1957) based on knowledge of the biosynthesis of the thymidylic acid component of DNA.

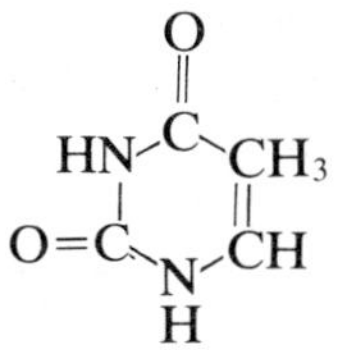

thymine

It was known that the methyl group of thymine is inserted into 2'-deoxyuridine-5'-phosphate by a series of reactions (the thymidylate synthetase system) catalysed by enzymes, and that this process might be interrupted by a substance with a stable fluorine substituted for hydrogen in the 5 position of uracil (fluorine containing analogues were known to be powerful metabolic poisons). It is administered intravenously or orally (absorption may be variable) and it can be applied topically in the form of a paste. Side effects include nausea, diarrhoea and vomiting, with some alopecia. Its toxic effects, which cannot be ameliorated by the administration of thymidine, include bone marrow depression and ulceration of the gastro-intestinal tract.

5-fluorouracil has been used in the palliation of inoperable tumours of the gastrointestinal tract and beneficial effects have been reported in advanced tumours of the bladder, cervix and ovary.

Cytosine arabinoside

Cytosine arabinoside is a combination of cytosine and the sugar arabinoside and it probably acts by inhibiting DNA polymerase rather than as a true pyrimidine analogue. Its principal use is in the treatment of acute myeloblastic leukaemia.

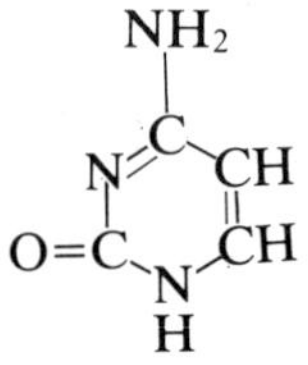

cytosine

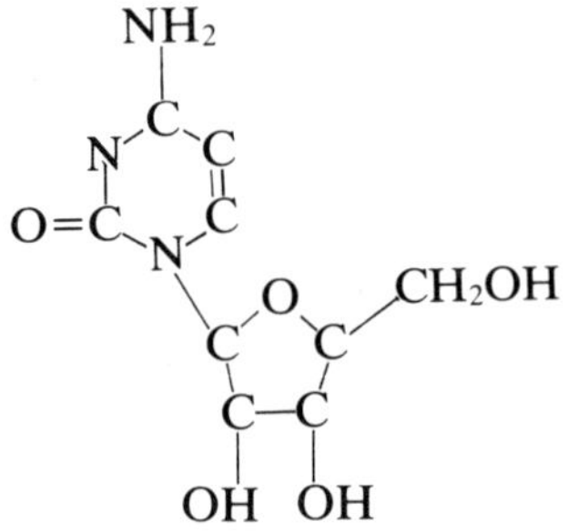

cytosine arabinoside

Vinca alkaloids

The periwinkle plant, *Catharanthus rosea* (*Vinca rosea*), was first drawn by John Miller and sent to the Chelsea Physic Garden, London, from Madagascar via the Jardin Des Plantes, Paris, and the drawing published August 29th, 1757. Its reputed medicinal properties led to an investigation, in 1949, of an alleged hypoglycaemic effect. Both the independent groups of Canadian scientists (Noble et al. 1958) and research workers at the laboratories of Eli Lilly and Co (Johnson et al. 1960) were unable to demonstrate hypoglycaemia in animals, but did show leukopoenia to such an extent that they used this property as a mark of the purification of an active alkaloid they called initially vincaleukoblastine—later shortened to vinblastine. Three other dimeric alkaloids containing both indole and dihydroindole were identified by fractionation: vincristine, vinleurosine and vinrosidine. Early antitumour activity was demonstrated against an acute lymphocytic leukaemia in mice.

Vinca alkaloids arrest mitotic division in metaphase by binding to the proteins of the microtubules involved in spindle formation, and like the anti-inflammatory agent colchicine and the antifungal agent griseofulvin, are referred to as 'spindle poisons' (Wilson et al. 1976).

High concentrations of vinca alkaloids have been shown to inhibit the inclusion of amino acids into transfer RNA (Creasey 1975).

Although similar in structure, vinblastine and vincristine have different anti-tumour activity spectra and toxicities. However, both are administered intra-venously and extravasation, especially of vincristine, causes intense irritation to the tissues, so severe in some cases that skin grafting the area affected may be required. The drugs disappear from the blood stream within an hour and are excreted via the liver into the bile. It has been shown that they enhance the accumulation of methotrexate in cultured tumour cells (Bender et al. 1975).

Vincristine R = CHO
Vinblastine R = CH$_3$

The dose limiting toxicity of vinblastine is bone marrow depression, although platelets may be selectively spared. Vincristine, on the other hand, causes little myelosuppression but much more neurotoxicity than vinblastine, mainly involving peripheral nerves. Reduced bowel motility, secondary to autonomic nerve involvement, is also common. Vincristine and vinblastine cause alopecia in about 20% of patients and like other cytotoxic agents which cause rapid destruction of tumour cell nuclei, hyperuricaemia may also occur, requiring the concomitant administration of allopurinol.

Vinblastine is used in combination drug therapy in the management of Hodgkin's disease, lymphoma, methotrexate resistant choriocarcinoma, and, in combination with bleomycin and cisplatin, produces remission in nearly all patients with advanced testicular teratoma (Einhorn and Donohue 1977).

Vincristine has been used in combination therapy in the management of acute lymphocytic and myelogenous leukaemia, advanced Hodgkin's disease, other lymphomas, Wilms's tumour, Ewing's and osteogenic sarcomas, also cancers of the breast and cervix.

Vindesine (deacetylvinblastine carboxyamide)

Vindesine was marketed as the first semisynthetic vinca alkaloid in 1980. It is currently undergoing evaluation and, to date, may be of use in the treatment of acute lymphoblastic leukaemia, blastic crises of chronic myeloid leukaemia and malignant melanoma resistant or unresponsive to other drug therapy.

Epipodophyllotoxin analogues

Podophyllotoxin is formed by the plant Podophyllum peltatum, known as the May apple or American mandrake. Podophyllin resin BP has been widely used for the topical treatment of plantar and perineal warts. Semisynthetic derivatives have been produced; VP16-213 and VM26 have undergone extensive clinical trials. A mention of these interesting agents is given after the Vinca alkaloids because they are similar to natural plant products and the parent compound, podophyllotoxin, functions as a spindle poison. However, later work has shown that etoposide (VP16-213) causes its major delay of cell cycle progression and its maximum cell killing in the S (DNA synthesis) and G_2 (RNA synthesis) phases (Issell and Crooke 1979).

At present etoposide is a very active single agent in the treatment of small cell bronchial carcinoma (Arnold 1979), and in combination with other drugs and surgery induces remission in more than half of patients with testicular teratoma resistant to other drugs (Williams et al. 1980).

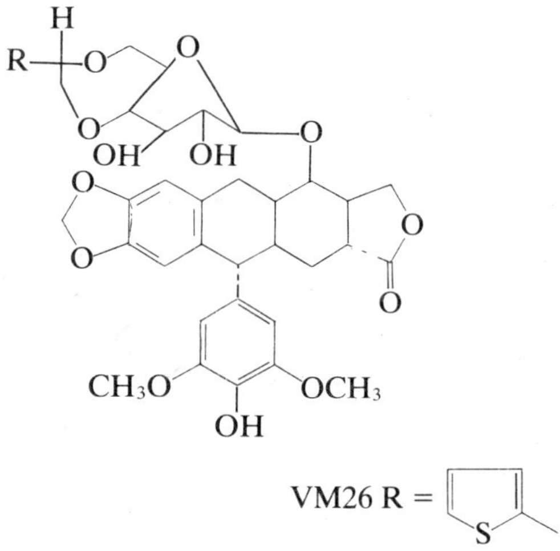

VM26 R =

VP16-213 R = CH_3

Antibiotics

Actinomycin D

A variety of antitumour antibiotics have been isolated from *Streptomyces* species and the first of these, Actinomycin A, was extracted from a culture broth of this soil organism in 1940 by Waksman and Woodruff, which was later shown to have inhibitory effects on the growth of sarcoma 180 in vivo in 1950. Actinomycin D, produced in 1954 (Vining and Waksman 1954) proved to be less toxic than the other actinomycins.

Actinomycin D binds to DNA in the presence of guanine and inhibits RNA synthesis. It is administered via a fast-flowing intravenous infusion as extravastion causes a severe local reaction, and the drug has a plasma half life of about 36 hours (Tattersall et al. 1975). It causes nausea, vomiting, malaise and marked myelo-suppression. Ulceration of the mouth and gastrointestinal tract is not uncommon; alopecia and acneiform skin lesions are seen in some patients. Actinomycin D can

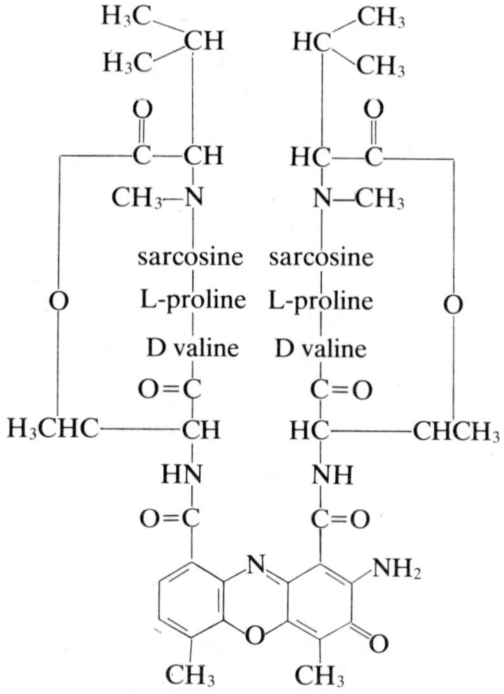

$$
\begin{array}{c}
\text{H}_3\text{C} \\
\quad\diagdown \text{CH} \qquad\qquad \text{HC}\diagup^{\text{CH}_3} \\
\text{H}_3\text{C}\diagup \qquad\qquad\qquad \diagdown \text{CH}_3
\end{array}
$$

structure of actinomycin D

H₃C—CH / H₃C (CH) ... HC—CH₃ / CH₃ (HC)

O ⸬ O
C—CH   HC—C
CH₃—N   N—CH₃

sarcosine   sarcosine
L-proline   L-proline
D valine   D valine
O=C   C=O
H₃CHC———CH   HC———CHCH₃
HN   NH
O=C   C=O

N

NH₂

O

O

CH₃   CH₃

actinomycin D

potentiate the effects of irradiation by inhibiting the repair of radiation-induced DNA damage and, if given after irradiation, can cause a reaction in the skin involved in the previous radiotherapy.

It is an immunosuppressive and has been used as such, but its cytotoxic properties, especially in combination with other agents such as vincristine and cyclophosphamide, are utilised in the treatment of several paediatric solid tumours, eg Wilms's tumour, Ewing's sarcoma and embryonal rhabdomyosarcoma. Actinomycin D is also effective in the treatment of methotrexate-resistant gestational choriocarcinoma (Lewis 1972).

Doxorubicin (Adriamycin)

Doxorubicin was introduced in the late 1960s following research performed in Italy (Arcamone et al. 1969). Again it is derived from a species of *Streptomyces*. It has a four-ringed structure linked via a glycosidic band to daunosamine, an amine sugar.

It acts by intercalating between base pairs of DNA (with local unwinding of the helical structure as the base pairs are moved apart) and inhibiting RNA synthesis by loss of template activity. Although active throughout the cell cycle, studies show more activity in the S phase than in the G_1 phase.

Doxorubicin (Adriamycin) is administered intravenously. Accidental extravasation causes intense tissue reaction and local necrosis. The majority of the drug

Doxorubicin R = OH
Daunorubicin R = H

is excreted via the biliary system—patients with reduced hepatic function may retain high levels. Side effects include nausea, vomiting and alopecia, the latter being universal and reversible when treatment is stopped. The initial report by Luce et al. (1973) that doxorubicin-related alopecia may be reduced by scalp cooling has led to various ice pack 'turbans' being used to prevent this distressing side effect and these have met with considerable success, although they are unpleasant to wear at the time. Bone marrow depression of a moderate degree is common but a more serious toxic effect is the development of cardiomyopathy, as the cardiac failure subsequently produced is usually refractory to the usual therapy. The chance of developing cardiotoxicity increases with the cumulative dose and stipulated maxima should not be exceeded (550 mg/m^2 is commonly recommended). Both mediastinal radiotherapy and high dose cyclophosphamide therapy also predispose to cardiotoxicity and concurrent doxorubicin dosage maximum is usually lowered to 450 mg/m^2 in such cases (Minnow et al. 1977).

Doxorubicin has shown activity in a wide range of solid tumours including cancers of the bladder, breast, ovary and cervix.

Daunorubicin
This drug is very similar in structure, mode of action, side effects and toxicity to doxorubicin. It has a different spectrum of activity, however, and its principal use is in the treatment of acute myeloblastic leukaemia.

Bleomycin
Introduced in the mid 1960s and reported from Japan (Umezawa et al. 1966) the bleomycins are water soluble glycopeptide antibiotics extracted from cultures of *Streptomyces verticillus* and is usually prepared as a mixture, about half of which is bleomycin A$_2$. It acts by causing fractures in single stranded DNA and inhibition of DNA synthesis, hence its effects on S and early G$_2$ phases. It is administered parenterally and is rapidly excreted into the urine. Side effects include oral mucositis, alopecia in 10–20% of patients, and pigmentation of the skin. Whilst

myelosuppression is surprisingly mild, bleomycin is toxic to the skin and lungs, resulting in basal infiltrates and interstitial pulmonary fibrosis, in about 10% of patients.

A total maximum dose of 200–300 mg is usually adhered to. The elderly, and patients who have been given previous radiotherapy, are especially susceptible to the pulmonary toxicity. Very severe anaphylactoid reactions are occasionally seen, especially in lymphoma patients.

It is popular for bleomycin to be used in the combination therapy (especially as it lacks serious myelotoxicity) of advanced testicular teratoma, squamous cell carcinoma of the head and neck, penis, vulva, and cervix, and in various types of lymphoma.

Mithramycin

Derived from *Streptomyces plicatus*, mithramycin inhibits RNA and DNA synthesis, especially the former. It is a toxic drug and is usually given over several hours to reduce gastrointestinal effects. It is used mainly in the treatment of testicular tumours and the management of hypercalcaemia. Its calcium lowering effects are thought to be due to inhibition of osteoclastic bone resorption.

Mitomycin C

Mitomycin C is also derived from *Streptomyces* species, and acts by interstrand cross linking and alkylating DNA. It is given intravenously and is highly vesicant. Delayed cumulative myelosuppression is frequently severe and dose limiting. Activity has been demonstrated in tumours of the breast, stomach and large bowel, pancreas, head and neck.

L-Aspariginase

Kidd (1953) reported the regression of transplanted subcutaneous lymphomas in mice and rats following the intraperitoneal injection of guinea pig serum, and that sera from rabbits and horses could not. A decade later, Broome (1963) showed that the antilymphoma effect was due to L-aspariginase and that some tumour cells have an important nutritional requirement for L-aspariginase. It is sometimes used in the management of acute leukaemia.

Hydroxyurea

Hydroxyurea inhibits the ribonucleotide reductases and thus prevents DNA synthesis. It is administered orally and has been used against a variety of cancers, eg malignant melanoma, head and neck tumours, but its use now is almost confined to the management of busulphan-resistant chronic myeloid leukaemia.

Procarbazine

Procarbazine is a derivative of hydrazine—originally synthesised as a potential monoamine oxidase inhibitor but was found to inhibit DNA and RNA synthesis. It is used in the treatment of Hodgkin's disease.

Dacarbazine

Dimethyl-triazino-imidazole carboxamide (DTIC) is used mainly in the treatment of malignant melanoma, some lymphomas and sarcomas. Its exact mode of action is not fully understood, but it appears to be similar to that of the alkylating agents.

Steroid hormones

Corticosteroids can interfere with DNA synthesis and occasionally find a place, although frequently without a great deal of clinical justification, in combination therapy regimens, especially in the treatment of leukaemias, lymphomas and breast cancers.

It was known from the late 1950s that target tissues of steroid hormones possess hormone specific receptors (Jensen and Jacobson 1962) and later on that

Table 7.1 Synopsis of side effects and major toxicities of cytotoxic agents used in the management of gynaecological malignancies

	Alopecia	Bladder	Gut	Heart	Kidney	Liver	Lung	Marrow	Nausea & vomiting	Periph nervous system	Skin	Veins
Actinomycin D	M		M					S	M		M	S
Adriamycin	S		M	S				M				S
Bleomycin	M		M				S		M	M	M	
Chlorambucil								M/S	M			
Cisplatin					S			M	S	M		
Cyclophosphamide	S	S	S					S	M			
5-Fluorouracil	M		M					M/S	M			
Hexamethylmelamine			M						M	M		
Melphalan								S	M			
Methotrexate	M		S			M		M/S	M			
Treosulphan								M/S				
Vinblastine	M							S				
Vincristine	M		M						S		S	

M = moderate
M/S = moderate severe
S = severe

progestational steroids lower the levels of oestrogen receptors in normal endometrium and endometrial tumours (Tseng and Gurpide 1975).

Kelley and Baker (1961) showed the effects of progestational steroids on advanced endometrial carcinoma and it has subsequently been shown that more than a third of such patients show evidence of response with prolonged survival following treatment with such substances as medroxyprogesterone acetate.

medroxyprogesterone acetate

References

Arcamone, F., Cassilnelli, G., Fantini, G., Grein, A., Orezzi, P., Poli, C., Spalla, C., Adriamycin: 14-hydroxy-daunomycin a new antitumour antibiotic from *S. peucetius* var. *carcins*. *Biotechnol. Bioeng.*, 1969, **11**, 1101.

Arnold, A. M., Podophyllotoxin derivative VP16-213. *Cancer Chemother. Pharmacol.*, 1979, **3**, 71–80.

Arnold, H., Bourseaux, F., Synthese und Abbau cytostatisch wirksamer cyclicher N-Phosphamidester des Bis (-chlora ethyl) amino. *Angew. Chem.*, 1958, **70**, 539–44.

Bagley, C. M., Bostick, F. W., De Vita, V. T., Clinical pharmacology of cyclophosphamide. *Cancer Res.*, 1973, **33**, 226.

Barker, G. H., Advances in Therapeutics. 1979, **1**, 19.

Barker, G. H., Controversies in Gynaecological Oncology. *Proceedings of the Royal College of Obstetrics and Gynaecology*, 1980, p. 129.

Barker, G. H., Wiltshaw, E., Randomised trial comparing low dose cisplatin and chlorambucil, with low dose cisplatin, chlorambucil and doxorubicin in advanced ovarian carcinoma. *Lancet*, 1981, **i**, 747–50.

Barker, G. H., Effects of cytotoxic drugs on fertility and pregnancy. In *Clinical Pharmacology in Obstetrics*, ed. P. J. Lewis, John Wright Ltd., 1982.

Bender, R. A., Bleyer, W. A., Frisby, S. A., Oliverio, V. T., Alteration of methotrexate uptake in human leukaemia cells by other agents. *Cancer Res.*, 1975, **35**, 1305.

Bergel, F., Stock, G. A., Cytotoxic alpha amino acids and peptides. *Brit. Empire Cancer Campaign*, 1953, **31**, 6–7.

Brock, N., Scheef, E., Ifosphamide—a new oxaz-phospharine compound. In *Proceedings of the 7th International Congress of Chemotherapy*, Prague, 1971 (Hejzlar, M., et al. Eds.) Munich, Urban and Schwarzenberg, 1972, 749–800.

Broome, J. D., Evidence that L-aspariginase of guinea pig serum is responsible for its antolymphoma effects. *J. Exptl. Med.*, 1963, **118**, 99.

Burchenal, J. H., Murphy, M. L., Ellison, R. R., Sykes, M. P., Tan, T. C., Leone, L. A., Karnofsky, D. A., Craver, L. F., Dargeon, H. W., Rhoads, C. P. *Blood*, 1953, **8**, 965.

Burnett, R., Leo Laboratories, personal communication, 1982.

Connors, T. A., Cox, P. J., Farmer, P. B., Foster, A. B., Jarman, M., Some studies of the active intermediates formed in the microsomal metabolism of cyclophosphamide and isophosphamide. *Biochem. Pharmacol.*, 1974, **23**, 115.

Creasey, W. A., Vinca alkaloids and colchicine. In *Antineoplastic and Immunosuppressive agents*, Part II, Ed. A. C. Sartorelli and D. G. Johns, Berlin, Springer Verlag, 1975, pp. 670–94.

Duschinsky, R., Pleven, E., Heidelberger, C. *J. Am. Chem. Soc.*, 1957, **79**, 4559.

Einhorn, L. H., Donohue, J., Cisdiammine dichloroplatinum, vinblastine and bleomycin combination chemotherapy in disseminated testicular cancer. *Ann. Int. Med.*, 1977, **87**, 293.

Elion, E. B., Burgi, E., Hitchings, G. H., Studies on condensed pyrimidine systems. IX. The synthesis of some substituted purines. *J. Am. Chem. Soc.*, 1952, **74**, 411–4.

Everett, J. L., Roberts, J. R., Ross, W. C. J., Aryl-2-halogenoalkylamines. Pt. XII. Some carboxylic derivatives of *NN*-di-2-chloroethylaniline. *J. Chem. Soc.* (Pt. III), 1953, 2386–92.

Farber, S., Diamond, L. K., Mercer, R. D., Sylvester, R. F., Woolf, V. A., Temporary remissions in acute leukaemia in children produced by folic acid antagonist 4-amethopteroyl glutamic acid (aminopterin). *New Engl. J. Med.*, 1948, **238**, 787–93.

Galton, D. A. G., Myeleran in chronic myeloid leukaemia: results of treatment. *Lancet*, 1953, **i**, 208–13.

Gilman, A., The initial clinical trial of nitrogen mustard. *Am. J. Surgery*, 1963, **105**, 574.

Haddow, A., Timmis, G. M., Bifunctional sulphonic acid esters with radiomimetic activity. *Acta Unio. Intern. contra Cancrum*, 1951, **7**, 469–71.

Haddow, A., Timmis, G. M., Brown, S. S., Tumour-inhibiting action of 1:6-dimethane sulphonyl-D-mannitol. *Nature*, 1958, **182**, 4643, p. 1164.

Hayes, D. M., Cvitkovic, E., Golbey, R. B., Scheiner, E., Helson, L., Krakoff, I. H., High dose cisplatinum diammine dichloride: Amelioration of renal toxicity by mannitol diuresis. *Cancer*, 1977, **39**, 1372.

Heere, J., Donnelly, S. T., Antitumour activity of hexamethylmelamine. *Proc. Am. Cancer Res.*, 1971, **12**, 101.

Issell, B. F., Crooke, S. T., Etoposide (VP16-213). *Cancer Treatment Reviews*, 1979, **6**, 107–24.

Jensen, E. V., Jacobson, H. I., Basic guides to the mechanisms of estrogenisation. *Rec. Prog. Hormone Res.*, 1962, **18**, 387–414.

Johnson, I. S., Wright, H. F., Svobode, G. H.,, Vlantis, J., Antitumour principles derived from Vinca rosea Linn. I., Vincaleukoblastine and leurosine. *Cancer Res.*, 1960, 20, 1016–22.

Kelley, R. M., Baker, W. H., Progestational agents in the treatment of carcinoma of the endometrium. *New Eng. Med. Jr.*, 1961, **264**, 216.

Khan, A., Hill, J. M., Grater, W., Loeb, E., MacLellan, A., Hill, N., Atopic hypersensitivity to cisdichlorodiammine platinum (II). *Cancer Res.*, 1975, **35**, 2766.

Kidd, J. G., Regression of transplanted lymphomas induced in vivo by means of normal guinea pig serum, 1. Course of transplanted cancers of various kinds of mice and rats given guinea pig serum, horse serum, or rabbit serum. *J. Exptl. Med.*, 1953, **98**, 565.

Legha, S. S., Slavik, M., Carter, S. K., Hexamethylmelamine: an evaluation of its role in the therapy of cancer. *Cancer*, 1976, **38**, 27.

Lewis, J. L., Chemotherapy of gestational choriocarcinoma. *Cancer*, 1972, **30**, 1517.

Li, M. C., Hertz, R., Spencer, D. B., Effect of methotrexate therapy on choriocarcinoma and chorioadenoma. *Proc. Soc. Expl. Biol. Med.*, 1956, **93**, 361.

Luce, J. K., Raffeto, T. J., Crisp, M., Grief, G. C., Prevention of alopecia by scalp cooling of patients receiving adriamycin. *Cancer Chemotherapy Rep.*, 1973, **57**, 108.

Minnow, R. A., Benjamin, R. S., Lee, E. T., Gottlieb, J. A., Adriamycin cardiomyopathy—risk factors. *Cancer*, 1977, **39**, 1397.

Noble, R. L., Beer, C. T., Cutts, J. H., Further biological activities of vincaleukoblastine—an alkaloid isolated from *Vinca rosea. Biochem. Pharmacol.*, 1958, **1**, 347–8.

Piel, I. J., Meyer, D., Perlia, C. P., Wolfe, V. I., Effects of cisdichlorodiammine platinum (II) (NSC–119875) on hearing function in man. *Cancer Chemother. Reports*, 1974, **58**, 871.

Rhoads, C. P., Karnofsky, D. A., Burchenal, J. H., Craver, L. F., Triethylene melamine in treatment of Hodgkin's disease and allied neoplasms. *Trans. Assoc. Am. Physicians*, 1950, **63**, 136–46.

Roberts, J. J., Pascoe, J. M., Cross linking of complimentary strands of DNA in mammalian cells by antitumour platinum compounds. *Nature*, 1972, **235**, 282.

Rodriguez, V., Bodley, G. P., Freireich, E. J., McCredie, K. B., McKelvey, E. M., Tashima, C. K., Reduction of ifosfamide toxicity using dose fractionisation. *Cancer Res.*, 1976, **36**, 2945–8.

Rosenberg, B., Van Camp, L., Krigas, T., Inhibition of cell division in Escherichia coli by electrolysis products from a platinum electrode. *Nature*, 1965, **205**, 698.

Rosenberg, B., Van Camp, L., Trosko, J. E., Mansour, V. H., Platinum compounds: A new class of potent antitumour agents. *Nature*, 1969, **222**, 385.

Rosenweig, M., Van Hoff, D., Slavik, M., Muggia, F., Cis-diammine dichloro-platinum(II). A new anticancer drug. *Ann. Intern. Med.*, 1977, **86** (6), 803–12.

Shay, H., Zarafonietis, C., Smith, N., Woldow, I., Sun, D. C. H., Treatment of leukaemia with thioTEPA. *A.M.A., Archs. Intern. Med.*, 1953, **92**, 628–45.

Tattersall, M. H. N., Sodergen, J. E., Sengupta, S. K., Trites, D. H., Modest, E. J., Frei, III E., Pharmokinetics of actinomycin D in patients with malignant melanoma. *Clin. Pharmacol. Ther.*, 1975, **17**, 701.

Trusheikina, V. I., Izuchenie proteinoopukhole-vogo deistviia sarkolizina na razlichnykh eksperimental 'nykh opukholiakh zhivotnykh = Carcinostatic effects of sarcolysin on various experimental tumours in animals. *Vopr. onkol., Leningrad*, 1956, **2**, 222–9.

Tseng, L., Gurpide, E., Effects of progestins on estradiol receptor levels in human endo-metrium. *J. Clin. Endocrinol. metabol.*, 1975, **41**, 402–4.

Umezawa, H., Maeda, K., Takeuchi, T., Okami, Y., New antibiotics, bleomycin A and B. *J. Antibiot.* (Tokyo), 1966, **19**, 200.

Van Dyk, J. J., Falkson, H. C., Van Der Merwe, A. M., Falkson, G., Unexpected toxicity in patients treated with iphosphamide. *Cancer Res.*, 1972, **32**, 921–4.

Vining, L. C., Waksman, S. A., Paper chromatographic identification of the actinomycins. *Science*, 1954, **120**, 389–92.

Waksman, S. A., Woodruff, H. B., Bacteriostatic and bacteriocidal substances produced by soil actinomyces. *Proc. Soc. Exptl. Biol. Med.*, 1940, **45**, 609.

Wasserman, T. H., Slavik, M., Carter, S. K., Clinical comparison of the nitrosoureas. *Cancer*, 1975, **36**, 1258.

Williams, S. D., Einhorn, L. H., Greco, F. A., Oldham, R., Fletcher, R., VP16-213 salvage therapy for refractory germinal neoplasm. *Cancer*, 1980, **46**, 2154–8.

Wilson, L., Anderson, K. A., Clein, D., Non stoichiometric poisoning of microtubule polymerization: A model for the mechanism of action of the vinca alkaloids, podophyllo-toxin and colchicine in *Cold Spring Harbor Conference on Cell Proliferation, III Cell Motility*, ed. by R. Goldman, T. Pollard, J. Rosenbaum, New York, Cold Spring Harbor Laboratory, 1976, pp. 1051–64.

Wiltshaw, E., Galton, D. A. G., Clinical effects of amino-acids carrying nitrogen mustard groups. In *Ciba Foundation Symposium on Amino Acids and Peptides with antimetabolic activity*, London, Little, Brown & Co., 1958, pp. 104–9.

Worzella, J. F., Kaiman, B. D., Johanson, B. M., Remirez, G., Bryan, G. T., Metabolism of hexamethylmelamine-ring-C_{14} in rats and man. *Cancer Res.*, 1974, **34**, 2669.

Wright, L. T., Wright, J. C., Prigot, A., Weintraub, S., *J. Natl. Med. Assoc.*, 1950, **42**, 343.

Chapter Eight

Effects of Cytotoxic Drugs on Fertility and the Fetus

Fertility

The question of subsequent fertility in young women being treated for cancer must not be dismissed. It may be uppermost in the mind of a patient, along with survival. Informed counselling before cytotoxic drugs are administered may well relieve considerable anxieties. Knowledge of the potential effects on fertility of cytotoxic drugs, the effects on the fetus when administered to pregnant women (for example, those in relapse from leukaemia) and potential carcinogenicity is gradually being accumulated. The author has reviewed this knowledge in more depth—see 'Cytotoxics in Pregnancy—effects on male and female fertility, carcinogenicity' in 'Clinical Pharmacology in Obstetrics' edited by Peter Lewis, published by John Wright Ltd., 1982, also 'The Long Term Sequelae of Cytotoxic Therapy' by A. Hilary Calvert, in *Cancer Topics*, Volume 3, Number 7, 1981, 77–9.

Radiotherapy, even at low doses, given to the ovaries will result in sterility. Many of the chemotherapeutic regimens involving high doses of alkylating agents produce gonadal failure in both men and women. Many modern cytotoxic regimens used in the treatment of cancer in younger patients have a reduced tendency to cause severe and permanent gonadal destruction. Chapman et al. (1979) showed that patients treated for Hodgkin's disease with mechlorethamine hydrochloride, vinblastine sulphate, procarbazine sulphate, procarbazine hydro-chloride and prednisone, developed ovarian failure in 49% of cases, 34% had failing function and only 17% had normal ovarian function. This led to irritability, irrationality and sexual withdrawal in many patients, with a high divorce rate. Hormone replacement therapy produced a dramatic relief of symptoms with great improvement in hot flushes, irritability, dyspareunia secondary to vaginal dryness and return of libido. Some clinicians recommend the use of oral contraceptives during chemotherapy, particularly for Hodgkin's Disease, to mask any symptoms of ovarian failure and possibly to protect the ovaries from the chemotherapy by putting the follicular elements at rest.

Use of non-alkylating agents, or alkylating agents in small doses, frequently leaves fertility preserved. After the treatment of chorionic carcinoma at Charing Cross Hospital, London, 1958–1978, 104 patients out of 611 died of their disease. Of 375 patients available for follow up, 177 conceived after chemotherapy, producing 315 pregnancies which resulted in 245 live births from 167 women, with 76 spontaneous or therapeutic abortions. Only five women wanting to conceive failed to do so. All who subsequently became pregnant had been treated with methotrexate whilst 40 were given cyclophosphamide and actinomycin D (Rustin et al. 1981).

Although there is obvious anxiety that gonadal damage produced by chemotherapy may lead to fetal abnormalities in subsequent pregnancies, this does not appear to be shown in practice. Cytotoxics given in pregnancy vary in their teratogenicity by a considerable degree. Animal experiments are largely misleading and conflicting results are obtained when comparing the influence of the same drug in pregnant laboratory animals and human beings.

Aminopterin and methotrexate are highly teratogenic if given in the first trimester of pregnancy. American studies showed that abortion was induced by the administration of such antifolates in about 50% of women and the rest invariably delivered a malformed fetus. Most of the reports concerning antifolates included remarks concerning the few numbers of fetal abnormalities which are produced when these drugs are given in the second and third trimesters—in direct contrast to the findings in animal experiments.

Women who have received cyclophosphamide in late pregnancy have produced normal infants. However, malformations have been reported; there is also an association with premature delivery (Schaison et al. 1979).

Although animal experiments with chlorambucil show that this alkylating agent is highly abortive and teratogenic, the risk in human beings appears to be nowhere near as great—'Quasi nul' as Schaison et al. (1979) state. In the offspring exposed to both chlorambucil and cyclophosphamide concern must be expressed over potential gonadal destruction.

The first pregnant woman to be given cisplatin was reported by Jacobs et al. (1980) in the treatment of an oat cell carcinoma of the cervix. Histological examination of the male fetus, including gonadal structures, appeared normal.

The administration of cytotoxic agents which are myelotoxic, such as cyclophosphamide, to pregnant women may well suppress the bone marrow of the fetus. Okun et al. (1979) describe a case of multiple chemotherapy given for maternal acute lymphoblastic leukaemia beginning in the twelfth week of pregnancy. Therapy resulted in sustained complete remission of the leukaemia and a live, normally developed infant was eventually delivered, but whose neonatal course was complicated by transient severe bone marrow hypoplasia.

Pizzuto et al. (1980), in Mexico, reported on six patients in whom acute leukaemia was diagnosed in pregnancy and three other pregnant women who were in remission from previously diagnosed leukaemia. Chemotherapy was given to seven patients during various trimesters of pregnancy. There was no evidence of congenital malformations in the offspring. Only one infant was pancytopoenic at birth.

Once again numerous malformations have been described following the use of vinca alkaloids in pregnant animals, but the teratogenic risk in humans appears low, and the same applies to the antibiotic cytotoxic drugs—actinomycin D, bleomycin, adriamycin (doxorubicin); Tobias and Bloom (1980), for example, not only reported treatment of two patients with doxorubicin (Adriamycin) in pregnancy without untoward effects on the fetus but mentioned three similarly successful cases in different parts of the world. The drug was, however, administered relatively late in the gestation.

Whilst overt teratogenic effects are not common, especially if the cytotoxic agents are given in the second and/or third trimesters of pregnancy (except the antifolates), Nicholson (1968) did point out that 40% of the normal infants born to his series of mothers receiving cytotoxic therapy in pregnancy were of low birth-weight for the period of gestation, compared to his findings of only 14% of 43 mothers with leukaemia who did not receive cytotoxic drugs who gave birth to underweight babies.

Carcinogenicity

The use of cytotoxic drugs in malignancies which achieve cure or prolonged survival, such as choriocarcinoma, has directed attention from beyond the immediate toxic effects to the long term problems these drugs may or may not produce. Since chemotherapy of cancer began with any significance around 30 years ago the long term effects are only gradually being documented now. Anecdotal reports abound in the literature but large numbers of long term follow-up patients are required before the long term sequalae of cytotoxic therapy can be identified with accuracy.

Cytotoxic drugs which act by alkylation are frequently carcinogenic in animals and possibly in man. Certain cytotoxics act as cocarcinogens in experimental systems and augment the carcinogenic potential of certain substances. Certain individuals may be more susceptible to the carcinogenicity than others. Age is a factor, with fetuses and infants at possible risk. The latency period between initial exposure to a normal carcinogen and clinical evidence of malignancy is prolonged in humans, not infrequently two to five decades. A contributory factor may be that most cytotoxic drugs depress immunological defences, since the synthesis of protein and nucleic acids is required for the metabolic changes in activating lymphocytes and macrophages in cell mediated immunity.

Dr Calvert (above) divides cytotoxic drugs into three groups: (i) carcinogens (ii) non-carcinogens (iii) possible carcinogens; examples being: (i) most alkylating agents, nitrosoureas (ii) mercaptopurine, methotrexate, vincristine (iii) doxo-rubicin (Adriamycin), bleomycin, cisplatin, fluorouracil. Cyclophosphamide, for instance, causes an increase of bladder cancers (Kinlen et al. 1980); chlorambucil is associated with the subsequent development of acute non-lymphocytic leukaemia and similar as are melphalan and treosulphan. Further information can be obtained from IARC 1975 Monograph on the evaluation of the carcinogenic risk of chemicals to man Volume 9, International Agency for Research on Cancer, Lyons.

References

Chapman, R. M., Sutcliffe, S. B., Malpas, J. S., Cytotoxic induced ovarian failure in women with Hodgkin's disease—effects on hormonal function. *JAMA*, 1979, **242**, 1877–81.

Jacobs, A. J., Marchevsky, A., Gordon, R. E., Deppe, G., Cohen, C. J., Oat cell carcinoma of the uterine cervix in a pregnant woman treated with cisdiammine-dichloroplatinum. *Gynaecologic Oncology*, 1980, **9**, 405–10.

Kinlen, L. J., Eastwood, J. B., Kerr, D. N. S., Moorhead, J. F., Oliver, D. O., Robinson, B. H. B., de Wardener, H. E., Wing, A. J., Cancer in patients receiving dialysis. *Brit. Med. Jr.*, 1980, **280**, 1401.

Nicholson, H. O., Cytotoxic drugs in pregnancy. *Jr. Obstet. Gynae. Brit. Commwth.*, 1968, **75**, 517–20.

Okun, D. B., Groncy, P. K., Sieger, L., Tanaka, K. R., Acute leukaemia in pregnancy. *Medical and Paediatric Oncology*, 1979, **7**, 315–9.

Pizzuto, J., Aviles, A., Noriega, L., Niz, J., Morales, M., Romero, F., Treatment of acute leukaemia during pregnancy: presentation of 9 cases. *Cancer Treat Rep.*, 1980, **64**, 679–83.

Rustin, G., Bagshawe, K. D., Newlands, E. S., Begent, R. H., Cytotoxic drugs and sterility. Letter, *Lancet*, 1981, **i**, 1316.

Schaison, G., Jacquillat, C., Auclerc, G., Weil, M., Les Risques foeto-embryonnaires des chimothérapies. *Bull. Cancer (Paris)*, 1979, **66** (2), 165–70.

Tobias, J. S., Bloom, H. J. G., Doxorubicin in Pregnancy. *Lancet*, 1980, **i**, 776.

Chapter Nine

Prediction of Response

Not every tumour is sensitive to every cytotoxic agent and, although drug regimens are chosen for each patient on the basis that her tumour is most likely to respond, clinicians would like to know, in every case, the answer to two fundamental questions: (1) is the individual tumour of the patient I am currently treating sensitive to the agent(s) I am giving? (2) if not, to what agents is it sensitive?

Attempts to answer these important questions have been provided by a variety of laboratory systems—none of these are as yet perfect but all are worthy of attention.

There are four broad areas of interest: drug challenges on: (i) cell suspensions (ii) cell colonies—clonogenic assays (iii) xenografts, in which human tumours are transplanted into suitably prepared laboratory animals (iv) spheroids.

In addition to providing a drug sensitivity screen for individual patients, rather like that for antimicrobial antibiotics, these systems offer a means of testing new cytotoxic agents before giving them to patients. This in vitro drug screening process is being organised by the National Cancer Institute in the USA using four computer linked centres testing 50 as yet uncoded new agents, which has led to the standardisation of techniques and improved quality control (Green 1982).

Cell suspension tests

There are a large number of in vitro short term assays to determine sensitivity or resistance of tumours to cytotoxic agents (Dendy 1976, Holmes and Little 1974, Knock et al. 1974, Wright and Walker 1975). Considerable interest was aroused by the highly predictive values produced by Salmon et al. (1978). However, serious doubts about the clinical value of such results have been expressed (Berenbaum 1974). A collaborative group in Germany, KSST (Cooperative Study group for Sensitivity testing of Tumours) involving nine different hospitals between 1975 and 1979 reported their results using a short term in vitro test (KSST 1981). Mechanically isolated tumour cells (500 000 per ml) were incubated with cytotoxic agents—4-hydroperoxycyclophosphamide and doxorubicin hydrochloride for three hours at 37°C. Radioactive labelled nucleic acid precursors, thymidine and uridine, were added during the last hour and cytotoxic agent uptake measured. These in vitro results were compared with the results of cytotoxic therapy in 155 patients, 72 of whom had ovarian carcinoma. The comparison between test and therapy results in untreated ovarian carcinoma stages III and IV were in agreement. In recurrent ovarian tumours none of those which were resistant in the test using doxorubicin responded clinically to chemotherapy. However, only 69% of all tumours thought to be sensitive during the test were found to be so clinically. Of ten patients with cervical carcinoma three were thought to be sensitive to doxorubicin on testing but after the patients were treated clinically there was no change in tumour size.

Cell colonies—clonogenic assays

Initial reports, such as those of Hamburger et al. (1978), gave the early impression that most human tumours could be grown in agar, after even the most crude cell separation procedures. Colonies of the vital stem (clonogenic) cells could be isolated and drug screens used on them. This is clearly not the case and the same groups are now reporting significant colony growth in only 30–40% of tumours depending upon the site (Green 1982); with adequate cell yields for in vitro drug testing down to 25% (Jones 1982).

However, whereas clinical applicability has not been as successful as hoped a large amount of information concerning cloning and tumour cell growth has been acquired enabling models for testing new anticancer drugs to be established.

Jones and his coworkers (1982), at the Institute of Cancer Research, in Surrey, England, have found, as have other groups, that those tumours which grow best in agar have often been obtained from patients who rapidly succumb to their disease, usually before a drug screen result can be obtained. It has become apparent that many of the so-called 'colonies' which the original investigators were counting were, in fact, plated clumps of cells. Many workers are now trying to improve plating efficiency and the success rate of direct cloning. The method of Courtenay and Mills (1978) is accepted as a highly creditable technique and their results have been corroborated by other workers in different centres, including that of the Cancer Research Fund Laboratories, London. Improvements in the media preparation, using serum free preparations, and the addition of growth factors are also being utilised (Green 1982). While the predictive accuracy of the current assays for resistance remains nearly 100% the predictive accuracy of sensitivity is probably about 55–60%— and cynics would put that at just above chance.

Nevertheless, direct cloning is currently being employed for Phase I and Phase II new drug screens and despite its obvious limitations it may be of some use—see Future Prospects, Chapter 22.

Xenografts

There have been many attempts to grow human tumours in other species. Peyrilhe in 1775 tried to implant a human tumour into a dog. Green transplanted tumours into the anterior chamber of the guinea-pig eye and workers in Boston in the 1950s implanted into the hamster cheek pouch, which affords protection against immune responses. At the same time Toolan established transplantable tumours in animals preconditioned using irradiation and cortisone. In the mid-1960s the role of the thymus gland derived lymphocytes in transplantation immunology was discovered leading to the preparation of recipient animals for xenografts, using a combination of thymectomy with antithymocyte serum or with irradiation and bone marrow reconstitution. Bone marrow reconstitution is now avoided by pretreatment of the recipient mice using cytosine arabinoside followed by 900R total body irradiation.

Congenitally athymic ('nude') mice have been used since the late 1960s, particularly in the USA. They accept a wide range of xenografts but are difficult to breed and sustain in large numbers.

Most gynaecological tumours are relatively successful in their ability to be xenografted—take rates vary between 20 and 50%. Xenografts often retain some of the characteristics of the source tumour eg the excretion of marker substances, hormone receptors, production of chachexia in the host mouse; other effects are changed. Xenografted tumours grow faster, on the whole, than the source tumour, but do not appear to have the same metastatic potential.

Although many authors have suggested that resistance or sensitivity of the source tumour to cytotoxic agents is mirrored by the xenograft eg using choriocarcinoma (Hayashi et al. 1978), it has not yet been conclusively shown that the response to therapy of a human tumour in a patient is reproduced when the same tumour is xenografted (Shorthouse et al. 1980). Similarly, response of xenografts to radiotherapy may be variable, perhaps because hypoxia may be determined as much by the mouse stroma as by the human tumour cells implanted (Steel and Peckham 1980). Davy et al. (1977) claimed a positive correlation between the effects of radiotherapy on ovarian carcinoma xenografts and actual patient response. Radiosensitisers, such as misonidazole, have also been effective in xenografts of human pancreatic carcinoma cells by workers at the Institute of Cancer Research, Surrey, England (Courtenay et al. 1978).

Two problems remain: (1) it takes several weeks or months to grow xenografted tumours ('passage' as it is known), treat the mouse with cytotoxic agents and then to observe their effects; and initial drug therapy cannot be withheld from the patient while results are obtained. (2) the pharmaco-dynamic problems of comparing the therapy of mice and humans.

Xenografted tumours may well play an important part in future screening programmes for new cytotoxic agents. For a fuller review of the whole subject of xenografting see Steel (1978), and Steel and Peckham (1980).

Spheroids

The multicellular spheroid (literally a thriving clump of tumour cells) first described by Sutherland et al. (1971), tries to bridge the gap between in vitro and in vivo tumour models. They are produced in suspension culture or by using a non-adherent coating on the tissue culture vessel. Monolayer formation is prevented and the tumour cells aggregate. Cell division then produces a sphere of cells capable of autonomous growth.

Jones (1981) points out that an obvious feature of the spheroid, not seen in the monolayer culture, is the three dimensional cell to cell contact which has an effect on cell repair ability after radiation damage and exposure to some cytotoxic drugs (Durand and Sutherland 1976, Twentyman 1980). Diffusion gradients also exist within the spheroid, as in the source tumour, and these may affect the distribution and effect of cytotoxic agents studied.

Preliminary results using spheroids obtained from patients directly, or via xenografts, indicate that measured growth delay in spheroids, including those of ovarian carcinoma, reflects clinical and xenograft chemosensitivity (Yuhas et al. 1979, Jones 1982).

The use of spheroids offers another laboratory model for the testing of cytotoxic agents both in screening and clinical use—their development will be observed with great interest.

References

Berenbaum, M. C., Predicting response of human cancer to chemotherapy. *Lancet*, 1974, **2**, 1141–2.

Courtenay, V. D., Mills, J., An in vitro colony assay for human tumours grown in immune-suppressed mice and treated in vivo with cytotoxic agents. *Br. J. Cancer*, 1978, **37**, 261.

Courtenay, V. D., Smith, I. E., Steel, G. G., The effect of misonidazole on the radiation response of clonogenic human pancreatic carcinoma cells. *Br. J. Cancer*, 1978, **37**, Suppl. III, 225.

Davy, M., Brustad, T., Mossige, J., Irradiation of human ovarian tumors in nude mice. *Proc. Second Int. Workshop on Nude Mice*, University of Tokyo Press, 1977, Stuttgart: Gustav Fischer Verlag.

Dendy, P., ed. Human tumours in short term culture. Techniques and clinical applications. London, New York, San Francisco: Academic Press, 1976.

Durand, R. E., Sutherland, R. M., Repair and reoxygenation following irradiation of an in vitro tumour model. *Int. J. Radiat. Oncol. Biol. Phys.*, 1976, **1**, 1119.

Green, J. A., Third Conference on Tumour Cloning, Tucson, Arizona. *Cancer Topics*, 1982, Vol. 3, No. 12, p. 140.

Hamburger, A. W., Salmon, S. E., Kim, M. B., Trent, J. M., Soehnlen, B. J., Alberts, D. S., Schmidt, H. J., Direct cloning of ovarian carcinoma cells in agar. *Cancer Res.*, 1978, **38**, 3438–43.

Hayashi, H., Kameya, T., Shimosato, Y., Mukojina, T., Chemotherapy of human chorio-carcinoma transplanted into nude mice. *Am. J. Obstet. Gynecol.*, 1978, **131**, 548.

Holmes, H. L., Little, J. M., Tissue-culture microtest for predicting response of human cancer to chemotherapy. *Lancet*, 1974, **2**, 985–7.

Jones, A. C., Human multicellular spheroids: an in vitro tumour model. *Cancer Topics*, 1981, Vol. 3, No. 8, Sept/Oct, p. 86.

Jones, A. C., personal communication, 1982.

Knock, F. E., Galt, R. M., Oester, Y. T., Sylvester, R., In vitro estimate of sensitivity of individual human tumors to antitumour agents: *Oncology*, 1974, **30**, 1–22.

KSST, In vitro short-term test to determine the resistance of human tumours to chemotherapy. *Cancer*, 1981, **48**, 2127–35.

Salmon, S. E., Hamburger, A. W., Soehnlein, B., Durie, B. G. M., Alberts, D. S., Moon, T. E., Quantification of differential sensitivity of human tumor stem cells to anticancer agents. *N. Engl. J. Med.*, 1978, **298**, 1321–7.

Shorthouse, A. J., Smyth, J. F., Steel, G. G., Ellison, M., Mills, J., Peckham, M. J., The human tumour xenograft—a valid model in experimental chemotherapy? *Br. J. Surg.*, 1980, **67**, 715.

Steel, G. G., The growth and therapeutic response of human tumours in immune-deficient mice. *Bull. Cancer*, 1978, **65**, 465.

Steel, G. G., Peckham, M. J., Human tumour xenografts: A critical appraisal. *Br. J. Cancer*, 1980, **41**, Suppl. IV, 133–41.

Sutherland, R. M., McCredie, J. A., Inch, W. R., Growth of multicell spheroids in tissue culture as a model of nodular carcinomas. *J. Natl. Cancer Inst.*, 1971, **46**, 113.

Twentyman, P. R., Response to chemotherapy of EMT6 spheroids as measured by growth delay and cell survival. *Br. J. Cancer*, 1980, **42**, 297.

Wright, J. C., Walker, D., A predictive test for the selection of cancer chemotherapeutic agents for the treatment of human cancer. *J. Surg. Oncol.*, 1975, **7**, 381–92.

Yuhas, J. M., Tarleton, A. E., Culo, F., Tumor line dependent interactions of irradiation and cisdiammine dichloro platinum in multicellular spheroid systems. *Int. J. Radiat. Oncol. Biol. Phys.*, 1979, **5**, 1373.

Chapter Ten

Carcinoma of the Ovary

Reference to ovarian carcinoma in this chapter is confined to serous and mucinous 'epithelial' ovarian tumours. Endometrioid, clear cell (mesonephroid) and Brenner tumours will be considered separately, along with the sex cord stromal tumours (granulosa, theca cell, androblastoma, gynandroblastoma) and the germ cell tumours (dysgerminoma, endodermal sinus tumour, embryonal carcinoma, choriocarcinoma, teratomas).

Ovarian carcinoma is the most common cause of death from gynaecological malignancy in the UK and USA. In 1978 there were 3765 deaths from the disease in England and Wales. Its incidence in the UK and the USA is about 11 per 100 000 and in Sweden 15 per 100 000. There are well-recognised associations between ovarian malignancy and breast carcinoma, low parity and relative infertility, and the author has reviewed further aetiological factors in the British Medical Journal (1979).

70% of patients present with advanced disease and this has an important influence on the chance of cure, which overall is only about one in three (see Table 10.1).

Women with such advanced disease who are untreated have a median survival of only nine months (Young 1975). The five year survival rate of women with advanced ovarian cancer treated with conventional (low dose) alkylating agents is only 0–9% (Barker 1981c).

Until recently comparison of results between different centres was compromised by the lack of universal staging systems. It is to be hoped that all centres are now using the FIGO system. Also the doses of chemotherapy used and the frequency of their administration in the past might be considered to be, in some cases, inadequate when compared to recent practices. For this reason only very recent trials are referred to in the rest of the discussion.

Table 10.1 Ovarian carcinoma

5 yr survival (Staging differs slightly from FIGO) in brackets

No. of patients	Stage I	II	III	IV
122	17 (72%)	59 (30%)	31 (3%)	15 (0%)

From the report by Dr V. M. Dalley of the Royal Marsden Hospital, London (1962)

Staging

From FIGO: International Federation of Gynaecology and Obstetrics (1976).

Stage Ia   growth limited to one ovary, no ascites
>   (i) no capsule penetration or rupture
>   (ii) capsule penetrated and/or ruptured

      Ib   growth limited to both ovaries, no ascites
>   (i) no capsule penetration or rupture
>   (ii) capsule penetrated or ruptured

      Ic   growth limited to one or both ovaries with ascites present, or malignant cells found in peritoneal washings

      IIa   growth involving one or both ovaries with extension and/or metastases to the uterus and/or tubes

      IIb   growth involving one or both ovaries with extension, direct or metastatic, to other pelvic tissues

      IIc   growth involving one or both ovaries with extension to other pelvic structures with ascites present or malignant cells found in the peritoneal washings

      III   growth involving one or both ovaries with intraperitoneal metastases outside the pelvis and/or positive retroperitoneal nodes

      IV   growth involving one or both ovaries with distant metastases. If pleural effusion is present the presence of malignant cells in the fluid must be confirmed

NB Intraperitoneal metastases on the surface of the liver are Stage III; parenchymal metastases are Stage IV.

Special Category: unexplored cases which are thought to be ovarian carcinoma.

Initial surgery: staging and tumour excision

An accurate description of the tumour burden—its size and extent—is essential, and should be made at laparotomy. Recommended preoperative investigations include blood counts, blood chemistry, liver function tests, chest X-rays, aspiration and cytological scrutiny of ascites and pleural effusions if present, excretion urography, barium enema to exclude bowel pathology, and ultrasonography.

The initial laparotomy should be performed in the knowledge that the peritoneal surfaces of the upper abdomen and the para-aortic nodes are frequent and early sites of metastases, along with invasion, directly or indirectly, of the omentum. A thorough inspection of the liver and subdiaphragmatic surfaces is mandatory, along with omentectomy to detect (and excise) occult disease in that organ. Any suspicious areas should be biopsied. Any peritoneal fluid should be sent to the cytology department along with peritoneal washings (usually of normal saline).

Having made a thorough survey, with biopsies, of the whole abdomen and pelvis all authors recommend the excision of all visible or palpable tumour. However, there is variance of opinion in deciding at what cost to the patient total excision should be achieved. From past studies the efficacy of subsequent chemotherapy is enhanced in the presence of very small amounts of residual tumour as compared to its effects in the presence of bulk residual disease (Young 1978), and of subsequent radiotherapy in the presence of minimal residual tumour (Dembo et al. 1979). The importance of adequate surgical staging cannot be over-emphasised but the need for extremely extensive surgical procedures, associated with high postoperative morbidity, eg stomas, may decline as modern chemotherapeutic agents become even more effective.

However, current opinion is that the removal of as much tumour as possible should be attempted at initial laparotomy (Griffiths 1975). The same American author later reported that the survival of patients with residual disease less than 1.5 cm in diameter was significantly better than those patients whose residual disease exceeded 1.5 cm (Griffiths and Fuller 1978).

Radiotherapy

Except for very early, well differentiated, epithelial tumours of the ovary, surgical management alone is seldom curative. The role of subsequent radiotherapy is currently undergoing re-evaluation. There appears to be little, if any, benefit in irradiating bulk disease and limited pelvic irradiation will not treat occult extrapelvic spread which is common in under-staged 'early' disease. Furthermore, the importance and frequency of spread of tumour along the paracolic gutters and through the diaphragm via the lymphatic system is now realised and the necessity of including the upper abdomen and lung bases becomes obvious. Using the 'moving strip' technique Dembo et al. (1979) in Toronto treated stages I, II and 'asymptomatic' stage III disease with total abdominal radiation (including the diaphragm) and demonstrated better survival in those patients, compared with patients treated with pelvic irradiation and a very small dose of chlorambucil—but only if total hysterectomy and bilateral salpingo-oophorectomy had been performed.

Smith and his colleagues in the USA (1975) reported that melphalan gave similar results in early cases of ovarian carcinoma with less morbidity. However, abdominal irradiation may have a place after successful treatment with chemotherapy as a means of eradicating residual tumour stem cells.

Early stage disease

30% of all patients will present with so-called 'early' disease ie stage I and II. Despite surgery and postoperative radiotherapy 70% of these patients will relapse within 5 years and require chemotherapy (Wiltshaw and Barker 1978). Rosenoff et al. (1975) laparoscoped 16 patients originally labelled as stage I or II and found that nearly half of them had diaphragmatic metastases and were obviously under-staged.

Recurrence rates of even the very earliest stages of the disease (Ia and Ib) are also alarming. Hreshchyshyn et al. (1978) reported a recurrence rate of 17% for patients receiving no treatment after surgery, 36% for patients treated with pelvic irradiation and 7% for patients given melphalan. Dembo et al. (1979) found that 5 year survival rates patients with stage Ib and II treated with total hysterectomy and bilateral salpingo-oophorectomy followed by pelvic irradiation were only 50%. Thus even early stages of ovarian cancer can prove lethal. Some prognostic indication in stage Ia may be given by the tumour grade as reported by Dembo et al. (1979) again.

In this Toronto series of 41 patients with stage Ia none of the 20 patients with well-differentiated carcinomas has had tumour relapse. However, there were five relapses amongst the remaining 21 patients with moderately or poorly differentiated carcinomas. Five of the well differentiated tumours had had cyst rupture. Four of the five relapses had received previous postoperative pelvic radiotherapy.

These authors concluded that observation alone is only appropriate in patients with well differentiated stage Ia tumours, whereas all other grades and stages merit postoperative therapy.

Ovarian cancer complicating pregnancy

Ovarian carcinoma is not common in pregnancy but it does offer an opportunity for early diagnosis since pregnant women undergo bimanual pelvic examinations and ultrasound scans in pregnancy. The incidence has been reported as 1:18 000 deliveries and 1:25 000 pregnancies—about 3% of all ovarian swellings discovered in pregnancy and explored at laparotomy (Fathalla 1972), ie lower than the malignancy rate in the non-pregnant.

Barber (1970) advises unilateral oophorectomy for stage Ia disease (negative peritoneal washings) and beyond this total hysterectomy, BSO, omentectomy and postoperative chemotherapy. Unilateral oophorectomy might be employed for dysgerminoma, granulosa thecal cell tumours, arrhenoblastomas, gynandroblastomas. If the patient has no wish for future fertility pelvic clearance is advised after the sixth postnatal week.

Chemotherapy of advanced disease

Initial attempts to manage patients with Stage III and IV, mostly inoperable, disease were encouraged by the responses achieved using single alkylating agents. Throughout the 1960s and 1970s various groups have endeavoured to evaluate the cytotoxic therapies with activity in ovarian cancer. As a broad generalisation it was found that the response rates in advanced disease to varying alkylating agents was about the same and that increasing their doses to very high levels, or combining alkylating agents, severely increased their toxicities without a vast improvement in either response rates or survival (Young et al. 1974).

Dr Wiltshaw at the Institute of Cancer Research and the Royal Marsden Hospital, London, reported in 1965 the results of patients treated with chlorambucil between 1958 and 1962. Of 72 cases of advanced disease 61% showed evidence of response and 25% were complete—remissions, with some notable exceptions, were relatively short—median 8 months, range 3 to 49 months. No second remissions were obtained despite the use of increased doses of chlorambucil or secondary treatment with cyclophosphamide, mannitol-myeleran or 6-mercaptopurine.

In the early 1970s a number of non-alkylating agents were also shown to exhibit some activity in ovarian cancer, eg doxorubicin (adriamycin) and hexamethylmelamine. In 1974 initial reports were made on the ability of cisplatin to initiate regression in advanced ovarian cancer (Wiltshaw and Carr 1974).

Table 10.2 gives an overall view of the very recent trials involving the initial treatment of advanced ovarian cancer using single agents. Earlier trials have been

Table 10.2   Use of single agents in the first line treatment of advanced ovarian carcinoma

Agent/Source	Evaluable patients	Response rates (%)	Median duration of remission (months)	Median survival (months)
Cyclophosphamide				
Bolis (1980)	33	42		13 (all)
Carmo-Pereira (1981)	29	62	10(CR + PR)	11 (all)
Edmonson (1979)	35	31		12 (all)
Izbicki (1977)	89	45	18(CR)	8 (all)
Melphalan				
Brodovsky (1977)	114	26		28(CR) 13(PR) 6(NR)
Creasman (1979)	63	29	6	12 (all)
Omura (1981)	64	38		12 (all)
Park (1980)	96	29	8(CR)	9 (all)
Piver (1978)	111	20		19(CR) 11(PR) 3(NR)
Smith (1975)	306	47		14 (all)
Trope (1981)	70	40		11 (all)
Turbow (1980)	23	30		14 (all)
Vogl (1981)	119	36		17 (all)
Young (1978)	37	54	25(CR)	17 (all)
Treosulphan				
Fennelly (1977)	25	60	9(CR + PR)	19(CR + PR) 7(NR)
White (1982)	31	74	17 + (CR)	21 + (CR) 12(PR) 9(NR)
Hexamethylmelamine				
Wharton (1979)	51	31		25(CR) 28(PR) 9(NR)
Adriamycin				
Smith (1978)	34	27		
Cisplatin				
100 mg/m^2 Wiltshaw (1981)	31	74		24(CR + PR) 12(NR)
90 mg/m^2 Gershenson (1981)	22	50		

criticised for their use of agents in what is now considered to be less than optimum doses and more modern methods of patient support, eg against myelosuppression (see pages 16 and 138), have allowed alkylating agents, in particular, to be given in relatively higher doses.

Table 10.3 Combination chemotherapy in the first line treatment of advanced ovarian carcinoma

Agent/Source	Evaluable patients	Response rates (%)	Median duration of remission (months)	Median survival (months)
Cyclophosphamide				
5-Fluorouracil				
Barlow (1980)	22	32	15 + (CR + PR)	15 (all)
Izbicki (1977)	29	69	18 (CR)	14 (all)
Cyclophosphamide				
5-Fluorouracil				
Methotrexate				
Brodovsky (1977)	110	41		17(CR) 9(PR) 5(NR)
Cyclophosphamide				
Methotrexate				
Barlow (1980)	21	67	15 + (CR + PR)	14 (all)
Cyclophosphamide				
Hexamethylmelamine				
Schwartz (1981)	20	50		14 (all)
Smith (1978)	32	40		
Cyclophosphamide				
Adriamycin				
Alberts (1979)	61	36	7 (CR + PR)	13 (all)
Bolis (1980)	33	52		14 (all)
Edmonson (1979)	36	36		12 (all)
Omura (1981a)	72	49		14 (all)
Schwartz (1981)	17	59		17 (all)
Turbow (1980)	24	71		14 (all)
Cyclophosphamide				
Adriamycin				
BCG vaccine				
Alberts (1979)	57	53	10 (CR + PR)	24 (all)
Cyclophosphamide				
Adriamycin				
5-Fluorouracil				
Aroney (1981)	16	62		18 + (CR + PR) 6(NR)
Cyclophosphamide				
Methotrexate				
5-Fluorouracil				
Hexamethylmelamine				
Carmo-Pereira (1981)	28	36	9 (CR + PR)	10 (all)
Neijt (1980)	23	52	22 + (CR) 8(PR)	22 + (CR)
Young (1978)	40	75	30 + (CR)	30 (all)

Table 10.3—continued

Agent/Source	Evaluable patients	Response rates (%)	Median duration of remission (months)	Median survival (months)
Melphalan *5-Fluorouracil* Park (1980)	77	27	14(CR)	14 (all)
Melphalan *5-Fluorouracil* *Methotrexate* Miller (1980)	57	40	21(CR + PR)	13 (all)
Melphalan *Hexamethylmelamine* Omura (1981a)	97	52		14 (all)
Melphalan *Adriamycin* Trope (1981)	72	63		17 (all)
Melphalan *Adriamycin* *5-Fluorouracil* Aroney (1981)				19(CR + PR) 9(NR)
Cisplatin *Cyclophosphamide* Decker (1980)	21			18 + (all)
Cisplatin *Adriamycin* Holland (1980)	48	74	15 + (CR + PR)	20 + (all)
Cisplatin *Chlorambucil* *±Adriamycin* Barker (1981a)	85	53	31 + (CR)	CR (not reached after 48) 9(PR) 9(NR)
Cisplatin *Adriamycin* *Cyclophosphamide* Ehrlich (1979) Einhorn (1981) Williams (1981)	35 56 35	69 80 80	26(CR) 16(PR)	CR (not reached after 24) 20 (all)
Cisplatin *Adriamycin* *Cyclophosphamide* *Hexamethylmelamine* Holland (1980) Vogl (1981)	36 127	80 50		19 (all)

Table 10.3 shows the recent results obtained using combination chemotherapy as first line treatment. Since all of the drugs quoted have had extensive phase I and II studies, ie their activity is clearly demonstrated already, the yardstick in the assessment of such therapy in advanced ovarian carcinoma must now be survival. However, survival data are often inadequate—results of trials are frequently reported too early to be able to offer any cogent comments on survival expectations. With some exceptions the overall impact of even combination therapy on 5 year survival rates has not been defined and longer term follow up is necessary. Hopefully the trials in progress at the moment at various centres throughout the world will provide this information.

It should be noted that median survival for stage III and IV non-responders to most therapy is about 7 months (Barker and Wiltshaw 1981, Fennelly 1977) and that this reflects the rapid course of untreated disease. The institution of cytotoxic therapy, therefore, should not be delayed but commenced as soon as possible after initial cytoreductive surgery. Wound healing in a patient receiving chemotherapy for the first time is rarely delayed and if effective treatment is given quickly the distressing reaccumulation of ascites and the regrowth of tumour masses can often be prevented.

Second line therapy

Ovarian cancer not responding, or becoming refractory to, initial alkylating agent therapy rarely responded to second line drug therapy (Stanhope et al. 1977); see Tables 10.4 and 10.5.

The ability of a small dose of cisplatin to produce a therapeutic response in patients suffering from refractory ovarian carcinoma was shown by Wiltshaw and Kroner (1976) and that the response rate appeared to be dose related. High dose cisplatin therapy was shown to produce an enhanced response rate (63%) with some patients in complete remission (18%) (Barker and Pring 1981c), and several of these patients enjoyed prolonged survival (greater than two years) including those who were rendered suitable for radical cytoreductive surgery at the end of their course of chemotherapy. Nevertheless, overall survival was short and relapse often occurred when therapy was discontinued (Barker and Wiltshaw 1981b) and it is reasonable to conclude that effective initial therapy is to be preferred rather than placing an unjustified reliance on second line 'salvage' type therapy which may well be unsuccessful even using agents which are highly active when used first line.

Routes of administration

Most chemotherapy for ovarian carcinoma is administered intravenously or orally. Occasional reports are made of other routes eg intraperitoneal, intrapleural. No convincing data are available to confirm any advantage in these other routes. Most drugs mentioned act via the blood stream, some even require activation in the liver, before reaching the tumour, and intraperitoneal and intrapleural drugs will normally enter the blood stream quickly and not act at a

Table 10.4   Use of single agents in the second line treatment of advanced ovarian carcinoma

Agent/Source	Evaluable patients	Response rates (%)	Median duration of remission (months)	Median survival (months)
Cyclophosphamide				
Miller (1980)	33	3		
Melphalan				
Stanhope (1977)	71	11		
Hexamethylmelamine				
Bolis (1979)	34	6	5(PR)	9(PR) 5(NR)
Bonomi (1979)	16	25	13(CR + PR)	21(CR + PR)
				9(NR)
Johnson (1979)	21	19	3(PR)	6(PR) 8(NR)
Omura (1981b)	39	21	4(CR + PR)	
Adriamycin				
Bolis (1978)	38	8		
Hubbard (1978)	18	0		3 (all)
O'Bryan (1973)	19	11		
Stanhope (1977)	27	0		
Cisplatin				
100 mg/m^2				
Barker (1981c)	86	63	8 + (CR)	
100 mg/m^2				
Pesando (1980)	32	34	6(CR + PR)	11(CR + PR)
				7(NR)
80 mg/m^2				
Williams (1979)	12	33		5 (all)
30–100 mg/m^2				
Young (1979)	161	25		
Treosulphan				
White (1982)	21	48	8(CR + PR)	13(CR + PR)
				5(NR)
CCNU/Me-CCNU				
Omura (1977)	57	0		
Etoposide (VP16)				
Maskens (1981)	18	0		
Radice (1979)	40	10		
Slayton (1979)	24	8	5 & 11 + (PR)	4 (all)
VM26				
Radice (1979)	20	40		
Samson (1978)	16	0		

local level. There seems, at the moment, little to be gained in subjecting the patient to alarming and potentially dangerous routes of administration.

It has been suggested that control of malignant pleural effusions and ascites might be better achieved by delivering cytotoxic agents into the pleural or peri-toneal cavities; however, if the tumour is sensitive to the agent(s) used, then

Table 10.5 Combination chemotherapy in the second line treatment of advanced ovarian carcinoma

Agent/Source	Evaluable patients	Response rates (%)	Median duration of remission (months)	Median survival (months)
Cyclophosphamide Actinomycin D 5-Fluorouracil Stanhope (1977)	145	6		
Cyclophosphamide Adriamycin Hexamethylmelamine Sessa (1981)	30	17	7(CR + PR)	11(CR + PR) 10(NR)
Cyclophosphamide Adriamycin 5-Fluorouracil C. parvum Rao (1977)	24	50		
Cyclophosphamide Methotrexate Vincristine Barlow (1979)	47	30	6(CR + PR)	10 + (CR + PR) 5(NR)
Cyclophosphamide Hexamethylmelamine Methotrexate 5-Fluorouracil Neijt (1980)	14	21	11(PR)	

Cisplatin (50 mg/m^2)
Adriamycin
  Briscoe (1978)
  Wallach (1980)
	20
	38
		35
		37
			4(CR + PR)	
				24 + (CR) 10(PR)

Cisplatin (50 mg/m^2) Adriamycin Cyclophosphamide Bruckner (1978)	24	50		9(CR + PR) 7 (all)
Cisplatin (50 mg/m^2) Adriamycin Hexamethylmelamine Vogl (1979)	27	67	7(CR + PR)	14 + (CR + PR) 8(NR)
Cisplatin (50 mg/m^2) Hexamethylmelamine 5-Fluorouracil Alberts (1980)	106	25	6(CR + PR)	9 (all)
Cisplatin (50 mg/m^2) Adriamycin Hexamethylmelamine 5-Fluorouracil Alberts (1980)	48	31	7(CR + PR)	9 (all)

Table 10.5—continued

Agent/Source	Evaluable patients	Response rates (%)	Median duration of remission (months)	Median survival (months)
Cisplatin (50 mg/m^2)				
Cyclophosphamide				
Hexamethylmelamine				
Adriamycin				
Kane (1979)	35	49	9(CR) 4(PR)	
Piver (1981)	20	0		4

pleural effusions and ascites will disappear after one or two courses of therapy—indeed, this is taken by many centres as a cardinal mark of response to therapy. There is, as yet, no acceptable evidence that the process is either hastened by intrapleural or intraperitoneal administration, or that tumours unresponsive to agents given orally or intravenously will subsequently respond to the same agents given into the pleural or peritoneal cavities. In addition, side effects and toxicity, eg nausea, myelosuppression, are not reduced.

Fibrosis-inducing agents, such as bleomycin, have been used to counteract malignant effusions, particularly pleural effusions secondary to breast carcinoma. Their success, if any, is limited. If fibrosis is induced in the pleural cavity, lung function is consequently reduced permanently, and residual pleural effusion frequently becomes loculated and difficult to aspirate subsequently. Any form of operative post-treatment assessment eg follow up laparoscopy, laparotomy, will be compromised or even contraindicated if fibrosis-inducing agents are instilled into the abdomen.

Patients with terminal disease in whom ascites or pleural effusions are causing discomfort and dyspnoea benefit from frequent, skilfully performed pleural aspirations and paracentesis abdominis. Fluid aspirated from the pleural cavities permits return of lung function until the reaccumulation of fluid a few weeks later, giving, at least, periods of relative comfort instead of permanent dyspnoea.

Tumour sensitivity

Several centres are endeavouring to produce a tumour cell sensitivity screen so that chemotherapy can be offered to patients with greater selectivity eg Hamburger et al. (1978) who claim to have been able to clone ovarian carcinoma cells consistently in agar against which drug challenges may be put. The University of Arizona team have also reported a 62% successful predictive assay for complete and partial remission and a 99% accuracy rate for the prediction of resistance (tumour colony growth being only 7 to 10 days) (Alberts et al. 1980). Ovarian tumours have been xenografted onto immune depressed mice for use in drug challenges and there is considerable interest in the use of spheroids—see Chapter 9.

However, these assays are, at present, of research interest only, but drug selectivity may be widespread in the future, thus saving time and drugs to ensure that each patient receives a drug to which her tumour is known to be sensitive. The effects of initial chemotherapy, given at present on a reasoned, but empirical choice, must be constantly reviewed in order to confirm response. If that confirmation is lacking, and the tumour appears to be unresponsive or progressing, then therapy should be changed or discontinued without delay.

Duration of treatment

Traditionally, treatment with alkylating agents was continued over several years or even for the remaining lifetime of the patient, without any substantial evidence to support such long term drug administration. Conversely, prolonged continuous treatment with alkylating agents is associated with an increased incidence of acute myeloblastic leukaemia in such patients and many clinicians are now reducing the duration of treatment and are giving intermittent therapy in which the leukaemic incidence is less.

Many potent combinations of chemotherapeutic agents currently in use have dose and duration limiting toxicities which often influence the time over which treatment is scheduled. Second look operative procedures may also be involved in the decision to discontinue therapy—see later, page 77.

Assessment of response

As mentioned in Chapter 3, it is essential to ensure that the tumour of each patient is showing adequate response to the selected chemotherapy as early as possible, and if the tumour is not responding then therapy should be changed or discontinued. Unnecessary chemotherapy may decrease marrow and other organ function so that subsequent, possibly effective, therapy may be compromised. With the effective schedules of therapy currently in use against ovarian cancer some evidence of response should be apparent after one or two courses of treatment. Despite widespread interest and research there is no tumour marker which can be totally relied upon either to confirm the diagnosis of ovarian carcinoma or to be used as an index of therapeutic efficacy, although some are proving of possible use—see Chapter 4.

At the Royal Marsden Hospital, London, Pussell et al. (1980) have shown that ultrasound scanning provides an accurate non-invasive means of assessing patients with advanced ovarian carcinoma and may be particularly accurate in the upper abdomen, liver, diaphragm and pelvis. Computerised axial tomography offers similar accuracy.

Tumours may be measured by ultrasonography and repeat scans, during chemotherapy schedules, may confirm response and tumour shrinkage, if present.

It is possible that nuclear magnetic resonance (NMR) properties may be helpful in the future in assessing patients initially and following tumour extent during chemotherapy since it has already been shown that NMR can distinguish malignant tissue from histologically negative tissue in cervix, myometrium and ovary in a cancer free patient or a patient with cancer in a different organ (Fruchter et al. 1978).

However, the final assessment of response is frequently made by an interval surgical procedure.

Second look surgery

Parks (1945) reported on three patients with ovarian carcinoma who had been treated with deep X-rays after initial laparotomy had revealed inoperable disease. The three then underwent a second laparotomy and subsequent tumour resection. Wangensteen (1949) is frequently given credit for popularising second look surgery but mainly in the management of large bowel cancers. For ovarian disease he advised reoperation in patients without clinical evidence of disease about 6 months after initial surgery and advised that residual or recurrent tumour was removed in its entirety. He also advocated a painstaking exploration to include multiple biopsies of all organs, peritoneum, nodes and suspicious areas.

Since then the rationale for performing second look surgery following chemotherapy for ovarian disease has been based on one or more of the following criteria:

(1) to assess response to therapy
(2) to plan the discontinuation of therapy
(3) resection of previously inoperable disease rendered operable by therapy
(4) complete surgical extirpation of any residual disease
(5) resection of disease previously considered inoperable by unfavourable factors such as the patient's clinical condition, inexperience of the surgeon, lack of suitable facilities and time etc.

1 Assessment of response to therapy

Subjective clinical assessment of response may well be inaccurate—Smith et al. (1976) found that 33% of 103 patients who underwent a second look laparotomy after chemotherapy and were thought to be in complete remission were found to have either stable or progressive disease. Longo and Young (1980) considered that only one half or one third of patients thought to have no further tumour at interval laparotomy would actually be free of disease.

As mentioned above, reliance upon purely clinical assessments of tumour response may successfully be replaced to a large extent by other modes of tumour quantification—eg by ultrasound scanning, computerised axial tomography, perhaps nuclear magnetic resonance scanning—but the final arbiter for many treatment programmes is an interval laparotomy. Macroscopic appearances may also be misleading as multiple biopsies taken from patients thought to be in complete remission may occasionally reveal tumour after histological scrutiny. In a series of second look laparotomies in such patients performed by Mr J. A. McKinna at the Royal Marsden Hospital, London, the author found that approximately 10% of patients who were found to have microscopic disease after multiple biopsies were, in fact, macroscopically clear of tumour at operation.

2 Discontinuation of therapy

There is no clear evidence to indicate the exact time span over which a course of treatment should be scheduled. In view of the toxicity and side effects modern chemotherapy for ovarian cancer creates and, bearing in mind the ever present risk of inducing leukaemia and other secondary malignancies in patients treated for prolonged periods with continuous alkylating agent therapy (Reimer et al. 1977), the duration of treatment should be as short as possible within the confines of safety from subsequent relapse—a guarantee of which is impossible to give, in the present state of our knowledge, even if treatment is continued for life. The safety margin is thus impossible to define. A proportion of patients declared clinically, macroscopically (at second look laparotomy) and histologically free of disease will subsequently relapse and die—presumably because tumour stem cells remain undetected, we know not where. However, it is prudent to continue therapy in a patient whose disease is obviously responding until at least there is no detectable tumour remaining and that the state of the disease may well be best evaluated by surgical means. This is the reason some authors advocate performing a second look laparotomy on women whose disease has obviously responded at intervals of 12 or even 18 months from the start of chemotherapy in an attempt to choose the best time to stop therapy.

3, 4 and 5 Further resection of tumour

Since many workers extol the value of the resection, completely if possible, of tumour at the primary operation it would be appropriate to re-operate as soon as possible on any patient who, for a variety of reasons, had a less than optimum primary procedure. In practice there is great reluctance to re-open such patients and chemotherapy is often commenced following poor surgical preparation. There are two possible solutions currently being examined: firstly, if patients have received less than adequate attempts at total resection of bulk disease at the initial operation they could be referred to a specialist gynaecological oncology department for immediate re-operation by more expert surgeons in more favourable conditions; secondly, surgeons performing the initial operation might be educated in the need for bulk resection which may require the attendance at the initial operation of a gynaecologist, gastro-enterological and urological surgeons—or a surgeon able to cope with all three specialities. During a recent survey in Belfast, the author was informed that 40% of patients with primary advanced ovarian cancer had their initial operations performed by general surgeons rather than gynaecologists with extensive oncological experience, and additional enquiries made by the author in other UK centres indicate that this is commonplace.

In the current light of our knowledge, there is every indication to ensure, by whatever means, that as much tumour as possible is removed, as quickly as possible, before initial chemotherapy is commenced. Having accepted this premise, the author cannot but remind readers, nevertheless, that of those chemotherapy regimens which could be regarded as successful in the treatment of solid tumours eg choriocarcinoma, testicular teratoma, Burkitt's lymphoma,

Hodgkin's disease, the extent of initial surgical resection does not make an indispensable contribution to cure and it is possible that future chemotherapy regimens will be sufficiently effective in many more tumours, including ovarian cancer, to obviate the need for extensive high morbidity primary surgery.

The value of secondary surgery in making contributions to survival length is highly questionable. Initial impressions at the Royal Marsden Hospital (Morgan et al. 1980) were that survival may be enhanced by interval tumour resection. Of 35 stage III and IV patients who underwent a second look laparotomy after six courses of low dose cisplatin, chlorambucil ± adriamycin, 10 patients were found to be free of disease, and a further 10 were rendered surgically free of disease. In 9 an incomplete but significant reduction in tumour mass was possible and in 6 patients only limited cytoreductive surgery was possible. In patients who failed to respond to therapy, and were unresectable, the median survival was 7.6 months; in patients who partially responded to therapy, and in whom surgical resection was incomplete, the median survival was 10 months; but in those in whom the surgical resection was complete at second look the median duration of survival was 32+ months.

Tepper et al. (1971) inferred from a small series that even if cure rates are not enhanced complete surgical removal of tumour at interval laparotomy can improve survival, 39 months compared to 20 months, in patients having had an incomplete resection and similar observations were made later by Frick et al. (1978).

The timing of such interval laparotomies is entirely arbitrary, as mentioned above, but if secondary tumour resection is a contribution of significance (the case is far from proven) it would seem sensible to perform this whilst the tumour is still responding to therapy rather than to wait until possible resistance to therapy develops. Suggestions from the M. D. Anderson Hospital and Tumour Institute (Smith et al. 1976) include the performance of a second look laparotomy might be appropriate after 12 months. Since the median survival of non-responders is only 7 months (Barker and Wiltshaw 1981a) candidates for a second operation after 12 months will be well selected, as they are potential long survivors. In units where inadequate primary surgery preponderates a shorter interval between first and second laparotomies might be indicated.

Among these difficult problems one thing is certain—there is a great need for carefully controlled, prospective, randomised trials to evaluate further the value, if any, of second look laparotomy.

Current thoughts concerning second look laparotomy technique

An extended vertical midline incision is commonly recommended and at opening the peritoneal cavity any fluid discovered should be carefully aspirated and sent for cytological scrutiny. If there is no fluid present, the paracolic gutters and pelvis should be irrigated with normal saline and the washings produced sent for evaluation to a cytologist experienced in this form of investigation. All peritoneal surfaces should be inspected, including the subsurfaces of the diaphragmatic cupolae. Views of this area may be improved by inserting a laparoscope through the vertical incision.

Lymph nodes, particularly the para-aortics, should be palpated carefully. The pelvis should be thoroughly searched and, in the author's experience, very early recurrence is often seen in the sites of resection of the ovarian pedicles and these should be identified for especial scrutiny. All macroscopic tumour should be removed in total if at all possible. If still present, the ovaries, tubes, uterus and omentum should be removed. All suspicious areas should be removed or biopsied. In particular adhesions should be resected and sent for histological analysis. The taking of peritoneal biopsies from all areas of the abdomen and pelvis is widely advocated in primary surgery (Day and Smith 1975), and in second look surgery, and even the removal of the peritoneum (Hudson 1981) is suggested. The value of this when balanced against the potential morbidity must be questioned, especially as tumour may lurk retroperitoneally—see later.

An in vivo inspection of the peritoneal surfaces using a special staining technique and a high-powered laparoscopic microscope, such as that advocated by Professor Kimiyama Oshkawa of the Nippon Medical School Tokyo, may yield still more information about the state of the disease than multiple blind biopsy.

Creasman et al. (1978) made the interesting suggestion that retroperitoneal fat might be the site of residual disease even when the intraperitoneal surfaces appear clear and advises the sampling of para-aortic fat.

Follow up laparoscopies

Bagley et al. (1973) pointed out that laparoscopy may frequently detect ovarian carcinoma metastatic to the diaphragm which is often missed at laparotomy, and laparoscopy has been used as second look procedure with relative safety and minimal morbidity (Quinn et al. 1980). Views may be limited by adhesions but, with the exception of the para-aortic nodes, nearly all suspicious areas can be biopsied and peritoneal washings taken.

Fifteen per cent of patients thought to be disease free following primary treatment of ovarian carcinoma were subsequently shown to have small deposits of disease and/or positive peritoneal washings in a series of laparoscopies at Chelsea Hospital for Women, London (Barker 1980).

Mangioni et al. (1979), whilst applauding the great value of this 'minor' surgery in the surveillance of patients having been treated successfully with chemotherapy in a 2½ year study, emphasised its limitations. 36% of patients whose laparoscopy was followed by laparotomy either immediately or within 10 days had their laparoscopic findings contradicted.

Immunotherapy

The effects of cancer of the ovaries or, indeed, any part of the body, on the immune system of a patient is the subject of intense research throughout the world. There remain many unanswered questions, including those concerned with carcinogenesis It is not surprising, therefore, that the attempts to manipulate the immune system therapeutically have been largely empirical and, to date, without widespread success.

The observation that intratumour injections of virus vaccines such as BCG could arrest the growth of metastases eg in malignant melanoma, encouraged further research into this phenomenon (Hunter-Craig et al. 1970, Sokal 1974). Similarly general stimulation of the immunoprotective mechanisms has been attempted by the injection of pyrogenic organisms eg *Corynebacterium parvum* (Israel and Halpern 1972). Such procedures have been incorporated into treatment schedules. Barlow et al. (1980), at Roswell Park Memorial Institute, Buffalo, New York, randomly allocated patients to receive or not non-specific immunotherapy with *C. parvum* to cyclophosphamide, methotrexate and 5-fluorouracil treatment for stage III and IV ovarian adenocarcinoma and concluded that the immunotherapy had no apparent effect on the chemo-therapeutic response.

Levamisole, a synthetic immunopotentiator (Haddsen 1975) has recently been under investigation but little of clinical value has been discovered to date. Trowbridge and Domingo (1981) have killed human tumour cells in vitro and inhibited their growth in vivo using a monoclonal antibody technique to produce an anti-transferrin receptor antibody linked to either Ricin A subunits or diphtheria fragment A, and both antibody conjugates inhibited protein synthesis in human leukaemic cells.

Order et al. (1981) at Johns Hopkins Oncology Center, Baltimore, in a series of experiments have endeavoured to improve their results of chemotherapy and radiotherapy in the management of ovarian cancer with an intraperitoneal administration of ovarian anticancer serum, prepared from human ovarian carcinoma cell extract injected into rabbits. It is not known whether this antiserum offers a therapeutic advantage.

Use of progestogens

From time to time there have been reports of short remissions occasionally induced in advanced or recurrent ovarian carcinoma following the use of pro-gestogens, especially in patients who have tumours included in the endometrioid type. Unfortunately, compared with carcinomas of the breast and endometrium the majority of ovarian tumours, even those of the endometrioid type, are relatively refractory to hormone manipulation of this nature.

Hiller (1960) reported that 15 mg tds of norethindrone had decreased the reaccumulation of ascites and malignant pleural effusions in an almost moribund sixty eight year old lady with advanced ovarian carcinoma which had not responded to forty treatments with radiotherapy and later radioactive chromium phosphate.

Jolles (1962) reported on ten patients with advanced ovarian tumours treated with concentrated hydroxyprogesterone capronate (Primolut Depot) out of which one had a good improvement with clearing of effusions from 3 to 6 months; three others had good tumour improvement and the rest nil improvement. Jolles also mentioned the increased appetite and sense of well being such patients enjoyed.

Of 8 patients treated by Varga and Henriksen in Los Angeles (1964) with 17-alpha-hydroxyprogesterone-17-n-caproate (Delalutin) two patients died after less than 4 days of therapy and only one of the remainder achieved a remission of short duration.

Kaufman (1966) using 17-alpha-hydroxy-6-alpha-methyl progesterone acetate = medroxy-progesterone acetate (Provera) induced an objective remission in one patient which lasted for 3 years. However, another ten patients failed to show any response.

Ward (1972) treated 29 patients with 17-alpha-hydroxy-19-norprogesterone 17-n-caproate (Depostat) out of which nine showed decreased re-accumulation of ascites/effusions and/or reduction in the size of abdominal masses over several months. A further 3 patients subjectively felt better despite advancing disease.

Malkasian et al. (1977), at the Mayo Clinic, treated 19 patients with medroxy-progesterone acetate. Of five patients who received 100 mg per day none had an objective response and one had her disease remain static for 4 months. Of the nine patients given 200 mg per day, one had an objective response for 4 months and two had their disease remain static for 4 and 5 months. Of the five who received 400 mg per day, none had an objective response and one had her disease remain static for 7 months.

References

Alberts, D. S., Moon, T. E., Stephens, R. A., Wilson, H., Oishi, N., Hilgers, R. D., O'Toole, R., Thigpen, J. T., Randomised study of chemoimmunotherapy for advanced ovarian carcinoma: a preliminary report of a Southwest Oncology Group. *Cancer Treat. Rep.*, 1979, **63**, 325–31.

Alberts, D. S., Chen, H. S. G., Soehnlen, B., Salmon, S. E., Surwit, E. A., Young, L., In vitro clonogenic assay for predicting response of ovarian cancer to chemotherapy. *Lancet*, 1980a, **2**, 34.

Alberts, D. S., Hilgers, R. D., Moon, T. E., O'Toole, R., Mantz, F., Martimbeau, P. W., Stephens, R. L., Rivkin, S., Mason, N., Cisplatin combination chemotherapy for drug resistant ovarian carcinoma. In: Prestayko, A. W., Crooke, S. T., eds. *Cisplatin: Current Status and New Developments*. New York: Academic Press, 1980, 392–401.

Aroney, R. S., Levi, J. A., Dalley, D. N., Triple drug chemotherapy for advanced ovarian carcinoma: comparative study of two regimens. *Med. J. Aust.*, 1981, **1**, 633–5.

Bagley, C. M., Jr., Young, R. C., Schein, P. S., Chabner, B. A., De Veita, V. T., Ovarian carcinoma metastatic to the diaphragm frequently undiagnosed at laparoscopy—a preliminary report. *Am. J. Obstet. Gynecol.*, 1973, **116**, 397–400.

Barber, H. K., Gynecological cancer complicating pregnancy. In *Gynecologic Oncology*, Excerpta Medica, Amsterdam, 1970.

Barker, G. H., Ovarian carcinoma—an opportunity for cure? In *Controversies in Gynaecological Oncology*, Proceedings of the Royal College of Obstetrics and Gynaecology, 1980, p. 124.

Barker, G. H., Wiltshaw, E., Randomised trial comparing low-dose cisplatin and chlorambucil with low-dose cisplatin, chlorambucil and doxorubicin in advanced ovarian carcinoma. *Lancet*, 1981a, **1**, 747–50.

Barker, G. H., Wiltshaw, E., Use of high dose cisdichloro-diammine platinum (II) (NSC-119875) following failure of previous chemotherapy for advanced carcinoma of the ovary. *Brit. Jr. Obs. Gynae.*, 1981b, **88**, 1192–9.

Barker, G. H., Pring, D. W., Advances in the management of ovarian cancer. *Update*, 1981c, 123–33.

Barlow, J. J., Piver, M. S., Second line efficacy of intermediate and high dose methotrexate with citrovorum factor rescue and cyclophosphamide in ovarian cancer. *Gynecol. Oncol.*, 1979, **7**, 233–8.

Barlow, J. J., Piver, M. S., Lele, S. B., High dose methotrexate with 'RESCUE' plus cyclophosphamide as initial chemotherapy in ovarian adenocarcinoma. A randomised trial with observations on the influence of C. parvum immunotherapy. *Cancer*, 1980, **46**, 1333–8.

Bolis, G., D'Incalci, M., Grammellini, F., Mangioni, C., Adriamycin in ovarian cancer patients resistant to cyclophosphamide. *Europ. J. Cancer*, 1978, **14**, 1401–6.

Bolis, G., D'Incalci, M., Mangioni, C., Belloni, C., Hexamethylmelamine in ovarian cancer resistant to cyclophosphamide and adriamycin. *Cancer Treat. Rep.*, 1979, **63**, 1375–7.

Bolis, G., Bortolozzi, G., Carinelli, G., D'Incalci, M., Gramellini, F., Morasca, L., Mangioni, C., Low dose cyclophosphamide in advanced ovarian cancer. *Cancer Chemother. Pharmacol.*, 1980, **4**, 129–32.

Bonomi, P. D., Mladineo, J., Morrin, B., Wilbanks, G., Slayton, R. E., Phase II trial of hexamethylmelamine in ovarian cancer resistant to alkylating agents. *Cancer Treat. Rep.*, 1979, **63**, 137–8.

Briscoe, K. E., Pasmantier, M. W., Ohnuma, T., Kennedy, B. J., Cis-dichlorodiammine platinum (II) and adriamycin treatment of advanced cancer. *Cancer Treat. Rep.*, 1978, **62**, 2027–30.

Br. Med. J., Editorial: Cancer of the ovary. 1979, **2**, 687–8.

Brodovsky, H. S., Temkin, N., Sears, M., Melphalan versus cyclophosphamide, methotrexate and 5-fluorouracil, in women with ovarian cancer. *Proc. Am. Soc. Clin. Oncol.*, 1977, **18**, 308.

Bruckner, H. W., Ratner, L. H., Cohen, C. J., Wallach, R., Kabakow, B., Greenspan, E. M., Holland, J. F., Combination chemotherapy for ovarian carcinoma with cyclophosphamide, adriamycin and cis-dichlorodiammine platinum (II) after failure of initial chemotherapy. *Cancer Treat. Rep.*, 1978, **62**, 1021–3.

Carmo-Pereira, J., Oliveira Costa, F., Henriques, E., Almeida Ricardo, J., Advanced ovarian carcinoma: A prospective and randomized clinical trial of cyclophosphamide versus combination cytotoxic therapy (Hexa CAF). *Cancer*, 1981, **48**, 1947–51.

Creasman, W. T., Abu-Ghazaleh, S., Schmidt, H. J., Retroperitoneal metastatic spread of ovarian cancer. *Gynecol. Oncol.*, 1978, **6**, 447–50.

Creasman, W. T., Gall, S. A., Blessing, J. A., Schmidt, H. J., Abu-Ghazaleh, S., Whisnant, J. K., DiSaia, P. J., Chemo-immunotherapy in the management of primary stage III ovarian cancer: a gynecologic oncology group study. *Cancer Treat. Rep.*, 1979, **63**, 319–23.

Dalley, V. M., Is preservation of the uterus worthwhile? *Amer. J. Roentgenol.*, 1962, **88**, 867–76.

Day, T. G., Smith, J. P., Diagnosis and staging of ovarian carcinoma. *Semin. Oncol.*, 1975, **3**, 217–22.

Decker, D. G., Fleming, T. R., Malkasian, G. C., Webb, M. J., Jefferies, J. A., Edmonson, J. H., Podratz, K. C., Gallenberg, M. M., A treatment programme for stage III and IV ovarian carcinoma – cyclophosphamide versus cyclophosphamide and cisplatin. *Gynecol. Oncol.* 1980, **10**, 368.

Dembo, A. J., Bush, R. S., Beale, F. A., Bean, H. A., Pringle, J. F., Sturgeon, J. F. G., The Princess Margaret Hospital Study of Ovarian Cancer Stages I, II and asymptomatic III presentations. *Cancer Treat. Rep.*, 1979, **63**, 249–54.

Edmonson, J. H., Fleming, T. R., Decker, D. G., Malkasian, G. D., Jorgensen, E. O., Jefferies, J. A., Webb, M. J., Kvols, L. K., Different chemotherapeutic sensitivities and host factors affecting prognosis in advanced ovarian carcinoma versus minimal residual disease. *Cancer Treat. Rep.*, 1979, **63**, 241–7.

Ehrlich, C. E., Einhorn, L., Williams, S. D., Morgan, J., Chemotherapy for Stage III–IV epithelial ovarian cancer with cis-dichlorodiammine platinum (II) adriamycin and cyclophosphamide. *Cancer Treat. Rep.*, 1979, **63**, 281–8.

Einhorn, L., Lecture. *Amer. Assoc. Cancer Res.*, 1981.

Fathalla, M. F., Factors in the causation and incidence of ovarian cancer. Obstetrical and Gynaecological Survey, 1972, **27**, 751–68.

Fennelly, J. J., Treosulphan in the management of ovarian carcinoma. *Br. J. Obstet. Gynae.*, 1977, **84**, 300–3.

Frick, G., Johnsson, J. E., Landberg, T., Snorradottir, M., Relaparotomy in advanced ovarian carcinoma. *Acta Obstet. Gynecol. Scand.*, 1978, **57**, 165–68.

Fruchter, R. G., Goldsmith, M., Boyce, J. G., Nicastri, A. D., Koutcher, J., Damadian, R., Nuclear magnetic resonance properties of gynaecological tissues. *Gynecologic Oncology*, 1978, **6**, 243–55.

Gershensen, D. M., Wharton, J. T., Herson, J., Edwards, C. L., Rutledge, F. N., Single agent cisplatinum therapy for advanced ovarian cancer. *Obstet. Gynecol.*, 1981, **58**, 487–96.

Griffiths, C. T., Surgical resection of tumour bulk in the primary treatment of ovarian carcinoma. *Symposium on Ovarian Carcinoma*, Natl. Cancer Inst. Monogr., 1975, **42**, 101–4.

Griffiths, C. T., Fuller, A. F., Intensive surgical and chemotherapeutic management of advanced ovarian cancer. *Surg. Clin. North Amer.*, 1978, **58**, 131–41.

Haddsen, J. W., Levamisole: A synthetic immunopotentiator under evaluation. *Sloan Kettering Memorial Cancer Center Clinical Bulletin*, 1975, **5**, 32.

Hamburger, A. W., Salmon, S. E., Kim, M. B., Trent, J. M., Soehlen, B. J., Alberts, D. S., Schmidt, H. J., Direct cloning of human ovarian carcinoma cells in agar. *Cancer Res.*, 1978, **38**, 3438–43.

Hiller, R. I., Norethindrone in the treatment of cancer. *J. of Abdominal Surgery*, 1960, 19–22.

Hooland, J. F., Bruckner, H. W., Cohen, C. J., Wallach, R. C., Gusberry, S. B., Greenspan, E. M., Goldberg, J., Cisplatin therapy of ovarian cancer. In: Prestayko, A. W., Crooke, S. T. (eds), *Cisplatin: Current status and New Developments*, New York: Academic Press, 1980, 383–91.

Hreshschyshyn, M. M., Norris, H. G., Park, R., et al., Postoperative treatment of resectable malignant and possibly malignant epithelial ovarian tumours with radiotherapy melphalan or no further therapy (Abstr. 9W57), *Proceedings of the 12th International Cancer Congress*, 1978, p. 157.

Hubbard, S. M., Barkes, P., Young, R. C., Adriamycin therapy for advanced ovarian carcinoma recurrent after chemotherapy. *Cancer Treat. Rep.*, 1978, **62**, 1375–7.

Hudson, C. N., Ovarian carcinoma—A gynaeological disorder? *Ann. R. Coll. Surg. Engl.*, 1981, **63**, 118–25.

Hunter-Craig, I., Newton, K. A., Westbury, G. et al., Use of vaccine virus in the treatment of metastatic malignant melanoma. *Br. Med. J.*, 1970, **2**, 512–13.

Israel, L., Halpern, B., Le corynebacterium parvum dans les cancers avances: Premiere évaluation de pactivité therapeutique de cette immuno-stimuline. *Nouv. Presse Med.*, 1972, **1**, 19–23.

Izbicki, R. M., Baker, R. L., Samson, M. K., McDonald, B., Vaitkevicius, V. K., 5 fluorouracil infusion and cyclophosphamide in the treatment of advanced ovarian cancer. *Cancer Treat. Rep.*, 1977, **61**, 1573–75.

Johnson, B. L., Fisher, R. I., Bender, R. A., DeVita, V., Chabner, B. A., Young, R. C., Hexamethylmelamine in alkylating agent-resistant ovarian carcinoma. *Cancer*, 1978, **42**, 2157–61.

Jolles, B., Progesterone in the treatment of advanced malignant tumours of the breast, ovary and uterus. *Br. J. Cancer*, 1962, **16**, 209–21.

Kane, R., Harvey, H., Andrews, T., Bernath, A., Curry, S., Dixon, R., Gottlieb, R., Kukrika, M., Lipton, A., Mortel, R., Ricci, J., White, D., Phase II trial of cyclophosphamide, hexamethylmelamine, adriamycin and cis-dichlorodiammine platinum

(II) combination chemotherapy in advanced ovarian carcinoma. *Cancer Treat. Rep.*, 1979, **63**, 307–9.

Kaufman, R. J. *Medical Clinics of North America*, 1966, **50**, 845.

Longo, D. L., Young, R. C. *Current treatment and new prospects. Therapeutic progress in ovarian cancer; testicular cancer, and sarcomas*, Boehavve Series Vol. 16, Ed. A. T. von Oosterom et al., Leiden, Univ. Press, pp. 61–76. 1980.

Malkasian, G. D., Decker, D. G., Jorgensen, E. O., Edmonson, J. H., Medroxy-progesterone acetate for the treatment of metastatic and recurrent ovarian carcinomata. *Cancer Treat. Rep.*, 1977, **61**, 913–14.

Mangioni, C., Bolis, G., Molteni, P., Belloni, C., Indications, advantages and limits of laparoscopy in ovarian cancer. *Gynecologic Oncology*, 1979, **7**, 47–55.

Maskens, A. P., Arnand, J. P., Lacave, A. J., De Jager, R. L., Hansen, H. H., Wolff, J., Phase II clinical trial of VP-16-213 in ovarian cancer. *Cancer Treat. Rep.*, 1981, **65**, 329–30.

Miller, A. B., Klaassen, D. J., Boyes, D. A., Dodds, D. J., Gerulath, A., Kirk, M. E., Levitt, M., Pearson, J. G., Wall, C., Combination versus sequential therapy with melphalan, 5-fluorouracil and methotrexate for advanced ovarian cancer. *Can. Med. Assoc. J.*, 1980, **123**, 365–71.

Morgan, M. W. E., Barker, G. H., Wiltshaw, E., McKinna, J. A., Second Look Operation in carcinoma of the ovary. *Clinical Oncology*, 1980, **6**, 292.

Neijt, J. P., van Lindert, A. C. M., Vendrik, C. P. J., Roozendaal, K. J., Struyvenberg, A., Linedo, H. M., Treatment of advanced ovarian carcinoma with a combination of hexa-methylmelamine, cyclophosphamide, methotrexate, and 5-fluorouracil (Hexa CAF) in patients with and without previous treatment. *Cancer Treat. Rep.*, 1980, **64**, 323–6.

O'Bryan, R. M., Luce, J. K., Talley, R. W., Gottlieb, J. A., Baker, L. H., Bonadonna, G., Phase II evaluation of adriamycin in human neoplasia. *Cancer*, 1973, **32**, 1–8.

Omura, G., Di Saia, O., Blessing, J., Boronow, R., Hreshschyshyn, M., Park, R., Chemotherapy for mustard-resistant ovarian carcinoma: a randomised trial of CCNU and methyl-CCNU. *Cancer Treat. Rep.*, 1977, **61**, 1533–5.

Omura, G. A., Blessing, J. A., Morrow, C. P., Buchsbaum, H. J., Homesley, H. D., Follow up on a randomised trial of melphalan plus hexamethylmelamine versus adriamycin plus cyclophosphamide in advanced ovarian adenocarcinoma. *Proc. Am. Soc. Clin. Oncol.*, 1981a, **22**, 470.

Omura, G. A., Greco, F. A., Birch, R., Hexamethylmelamine in mustard-resistant ovarian adenocarcinoma. *Cancer Treat. Rep.*, 1981b, **65**, 530–1.

Order, S. E., Rosenshein, N., Klein, J. L., Leibel, S., Pino Y Torres, J., Ettinger, D., The integration of new therapies and radiation in the management of ovarian cancer. *Cancer*, 1981, **48**, 590–6.

Park, R. C., Blom, J., Di Saia, O., Lagasse, L. D., Blessing, J. A., Treatment of women with disseminated or recurrent advanced ovarian cancer with melphalan alone, in combination with 5-fluorouracil and dactinomycin, or with the combination of cytoxan, 5-fluorouracil and dactinomycin. *Cancer*, 1980, **45**, 2529–42.

Parks, T. J., Carcinoma of the ovary treated preoperatively with deep X-rays; report of three cases. *Am. J. Obstet. Gynecol.*, 1945, **49**, 676–85.

Pessando, J. M., Come, S. E., Stark, J., Parker, L. M., Griffiths, C. T., Cannellos, G. P., Cis diamminedichloro platinum (II) therapy for advanced ovarian cancer. *Cancer Treat. Rep.*, 1980, **64**, 1147–8.

Piver, M. S., Barlow, J. J., Pazigi, R., Blumenson, L. E., Melphalan chemotherapy in advanced ovarian carcinoma. *Obstet. Gynecol.*, 1978, **51**, 352–6.

Piver, M. S., Lele, S., Barlow, J. J., Cyclophosphamide, hexamethylmelamine, doxo-rubicin and cisplatin (CHAD) as second line chemotherapy for ovarian carcinoma. *Cancer Treat. Rep.*, 1981, **65**, 149–51.

Pussell, S. J., Cosgrove, D. O., Hinton, J., Wiltshaw, E., Barker, G. H., Carcinoma of the ovary: correlation of ultrasound with second-look laparotomy. *Brit. J. Obstet. Gynae.*, 1980, **87**, 1140–4.

Quinn, M. A., Bishop, G. J., Campbell, J. J., Rodgerson, J., Pepperell, R. J., Laparoscopic follow up of patients with ovarian carcinoma. *Br. J. Obstet. Gynae.*, 1980, **87**, 1132–9.

Radice, P. A., Bunn, P. A., Jr., Ihde, D. C., Therapeutic trials with VP-16-213 and VM-26: active agents in small cell lung cancer, non-Hodgkin's lymphomata and other malignancies. *Cancer Treat. Rep.*, 1979, **63**, 1231–40.

Rao, B., Wanebo, H. J., Ochoa, M., Lewis, J. L., Oettgen, H., Intravenous Corynebacterium parvum. An adjustment to chemotherapy for resistant advanced ovarian cancer. *Cancer*, 1977, **39**, 514–26.

Reimer, R. R., Hoover, R., Fraumeni, J. F., Young, R. C., Acute leukaemia after alkylating agent therapy of ovarian cancer. *N. Engl. Med. J.*, 1977, **297**, 177–81.

Rosenoff, S. H., De Vita, V. T., Hubbard, S., Young, R. C., Peritoneoscopy in the staging and follow up of ovarian cancer. *Semin. Oncol.*, 1975, **2**, 223–8.

Samson, M. K., Baker, L. H., Talley, R. W., Fraile, R. J., VM 26: a clinical study in advanced cancer of the lung and ovary. *Eur. J. Cancer*, 1978, **14**, 1395–9.

Schwartz, P. E., Lawrence, R., Katz, M., Combination chemotherapy for advanced ovarian cancer: a prospective randomised trial comparing hexamethylmelamine and cyclophosphamide to doxorubicin and cyclophosphamide. *Cancer Treat. Rep.*, 1981, **65**, 137–41.

Sessa, C., Bolis, G., Valente, I., Mangioni, C., Hexamethylmelamine doxorubicin and cyclophosphamide in advanced ovarian cancer resistant to previous chemotherapy. *Cancer Treat. Rep.*, 1981, **65**, 172–3.

Slayton, R. E., Creasman, W. T., Petty, W., Bundy, B., Blessing, J. A., Phase II trial of VP-16-213 in the treatment of advanced squamous cell carcinoma of the cervix and adenocarcinomas of the ovary: a Gynecologic Oncology Group Study. *Cancer Treat. Rep.*, 1979, **63**, 2089–91.

Smith, J. P., Rutledge, F. N., Declas, L., Results of chemotherapy as an adjunct to surgery in patients with localised ovarian cancer. *Semin. Oncol.*, 1975a, **2**, 277–82.

Smith, J. P., Rutledge, F. N., Chemotherapy of advanced ovarian cancer. *N.C.I. Monograph*, 1975b, **42**, 141–3.

Smith, J. P., Delgado, G., Rutledge, F., Second look operations in ovarian carcinoma—post chemotherapy. *Cancer*, 1976, **38**, 1438–42.

Smith, J. P., Chemotherapy in gynecologic cancer. *Surg. Clin. North Am.*, 1978, **581**, 201–15.

Sokal, J. E., Aungst, C. W., Snyderman, M., Delay in progression of malignant lymphoma after BCG vaccination. *N. Engl. J. Med.*, 1974, **291**, 1226–30.

Stanhope, C. R., Smith, J. P., Rutledge, F., Second trial drugs in ovarian cancer. *Gynecol. Oncol.*, 1977, **5**, 52–8.

Tepper, E., Sanfilippo, L. J., Gray, J., Second look surgery after radiation therapy for advanced stage carcinoma of the ovary. *Am. J. Roentgenol.*, 1971, **112**, 755–9.

Trope, C., A prospective and randomised trial comparison of melphalan versus adriamycin and melphalan in advanced ovarian carcinoma. *Proc. Amer. Soc. Clin. On.*, 1981, **22**, 469.

Trowbridge, I., Domingo, D., Antitransferrin receptor monoclonal antibody and toxin-antibody conjugates affect growth of human tumour cells. *Nature*, 1981, **294**, 171.

Turbow, M. M., Jones, H., Yu, V. K., Greenberg, B., Hannigan, J., Torti, F. M., Chemotherapy of ovarian carcinoma: a comparison of melphalan vs. adriamycin-cyclophosphamide. *Proc. Am. Assoc. Cancer Res.*, 1980, **21**, 196.

Varga, A., Henriksen, E., Effect of 17-alpha-hydroxyprogesterone 17-n-caproate on various pelvic malignancies. *Obstet. Gynecol.*, 1964, **23**, 51–2.

Vogl, S. E., Berenzweig, M., Kaplan, B. H., Moukhtar, M., Bulkin, W., The CHAD and HAD regimens in advanced ovarian cancer: combination chemotherapy including cyclophosphamide, hexamethylmelamine, adriamycin and cis-dichlorodiammine platinum (II). *Cancer Treat. Rep.*, 1979, **63**, 311–17.

Vogl, S. E., Pagano, M., Kaplan, B., Cyclophosphamide, hexamethylmelamine, adriamycin and cisplatin versus melphalan for advanced ovarian cancer. *Proc. Amer. Soc. Clin. Onc.*, 1981, **22**, 469.

Wallach, R. C., Cohen, C., Bruckner, H., Kabokow, B., Deppe, G., Ratner, L., Chemotherapy of recurrent ovarian carcinoma with cis-dichlorodiammine platinum (II) and adriamycin. *Obstet. Gynecol.*, 1980, **55**, 371–2.

Wangensteen, O. H., Cancer of the colon and rectum: with special reference to (1) earlier recognition of alimentary tract malignancy (2) secondary delayed re-entry of the abdomen in patients exhibiting lymph node involvement (3) subtotal primary excision of the colon (4) operation in obstruction. *Wis. Med. J.*, 1949, **48**, 591.

Ward, H. W. C., Progestogen therapy for ovarian carcinoma. *J. Obstet. Gynaecol. of the Brit. Commwlth.*, 1972, **79**, 555–9.

Wharton, J. T., Rutledge, F., Smith, J. P., Herson, J., Hodge, M. P., Hexamethylmelamine: an evaluation of its role in the treatment of ovarian cancer. *Am. J. Obstet. Gynecol.*, 1979, **133**, 833–44.

White, W. F., Continuous versus intermittent treatment with treosulphan in advanced ovarian cancer. 1982, *Curr. Chemother.* (in press).

Williams, C. J., Stevenson, K. E., Buchanan, R. B., Whitehouse, J. M. A., Advanced ovarian carcinoma: a pilot study of cis-dichlorodiammine platinum (II) in combination with adriamycin and cyclophosphamide in previously untreated patients and as a single agent in previously treated patients. *Cancer Treat. Rep.*, 1979, **63**, 1745–53.

Williams, C., Mead, G., Arnold, A., Green, J., Buchanan, R., Whitehouse, J., Platinum based chemotherapy of advanced ovarian carcinoma. *UICC Conference on Clinical Oncology and 7th Annual Meeting of the European Society for Medical Oncology*, 28–31 Oct. 1981, Lausanne, Switzerland, p. 106, Abstract 12–0190.

Wiltshaw, E., Chlorambucil in the treatment of primary adenocarcinoma of the ovary. *Br. J. Obstet. Gynae.*, 1965, **72**, 586–94.

Wiltshaw, E., Carr, B., Cisplatinum II diamminedichloride: clinical experience of the Royal Marsden Hospital and Institute of Cancer Research, London. *Recent Results in Cancer Research*, 1974, **48**, 178–82.

Wiltshaw, E., Kroner, T., Phase II study of cis-dichloro-diammine platinum (II) in advanced adenocarcinoma of the ovary. *Cancer Treat. Rep.*, 1976, **60**, 55–60.

Wiltshaw, E., Barker, G. H. *Biochemie*, 1978, **60**, 925.

Wiltshaw, E., Kankipata, S. R., Barker, G. H., A prospective randomised study of cisplatinum as a single agent and in combination with chlorambucil in advanced ovarian carcinoma. *BACR* 22nd AGM University of Keele, April 1981, to be published.

Young, R. C., Canellos, G. P., Chabner, B. A., et al., Chemotherapy of advanced ovarian carcinoma. A prospective randomised comparison of phenylalanine mustard and high dose cyclophosphamide. *Gynecol. Oncol.*, 1974, **2**, 480–97.

Young, R. C., Chemotherapy of ovarian cancer: Past and present. *Semin. Oncol.*, 1975, **2**, 267.

Young, R. C., Chabner, B. A., Hubbard, S. P., Fisher, R. I., Bender, R. A., Anderson, T., Simon, R. M., Canellos, G. P., De Vita, V. T., Advanced ovarian adenocarcinoma. A prospective clinical trial of melphalan (L-PAM) versus combination chemotherapy. *N. Engl. J. Med.*, 1978, **299**, 1261–6.

Young, R. C., Von Hoff, D. D., Gormley, P., Makuch, R., Cassidy, J., Howser, D., Bull, J. M., Cis-dichlorodiammine platinum (II) for the treatment of advanced ovarian cancer. *Cancer Treat. Rep.*, 1979, **63**, 1539–44.

Chapter Eleven

Sex Cord Stromal Cell Tumours

Granulosa and theca cell tumours of the ovary

The name granulosa cell tumour was initially coined by von Werdt in 1914 (Busby and Anderson 1954) although the tumour 'adenoma of the Graafian follicles' was described by von Kahldon in 1895, and earlier by Rokitansky in 1859.

Björkholm and Silfverswärd (1980) analysed 936 women with granulosa and theca cell tumours between 1958 and 1972 in Sweden and found a crude incidence of 0.72 and 0.74 respectively per 100 000 of the female population unchanged during the time interval. Incidence rates increased almost linearly from 35 to 69 years. The women displayed an increased risk of developing endometrial carcinoma and malignant lymphoma, and also possibly breast, colon and thyroid carcinoma.

Histological review of the endometrium in 147 cases from the Mayo clinic (Evans et al. 1980) revealed that hyperplasia was more frequent in patients with granulosa cell tumours than theca cell tumours (55% versus 37%) whereas adenocarcinoma was more prevalent in theca cell tumours (27% versus 13%). Adenocarcinoma of the endometrium associated thus was well differentiated in all cases, with no greater than superficial invasion (5 mm or less).

Björkholm and Patterson (1980) reported on the results of treatment in 305 patients with granulosa, theca and mixed tumour: 225 received surgery and radiotherapy and 53 surgery only. None of the thecoma patients, but 21% of the granulosa cell tumour patients, died of their disease. The five-year survival for granulosa cell tumour patients of all stages was 85%.

Recurrence of granulosa cell tumour may be after considerable periods of time. Laczkovics (1977) reported on a patient in whom a granulosa cell tumour of the right ovary was removed at 47 years of age. Fourteen years later the same type of tumour was found in the left ovary together with an adenocarcinoma of the endometrium. Five years after removal of these tumours splenectomy was performed to remove metastases. Fox et al. (1975) pointed out that because of the long natural history of many granulosa cell tumours, crude death rates over a relatively short period give little indication of the true malignant potential of these cancers and showed that if no patient died from any other disease, approximately half of them would die as a result of their tumour within 20 years.

Lusch et al. (1978) indicated that granulosa cell tumours represent 0.6 to 4.6% of ovarian neoplasms and that 20 to 30% of patients die from late recurrences.

Pankratz et al. (1978) followed up 61 patients (1944–1974) with granulosa cell tumours in British Columbia and found that though the 5 year survival rate was 78%, the 15 year rate fell to 50%.

The mean time from diagnosis to death in 42 out of 198 women in Sweden who died from granulosa cell tumour was 10.5 years (Björkholm and Silfverswärd 1981), median 7.5 years (range 1 to 30 years). They emphasised that tumour rupture at operation is associated with a poor prognosis, as is advanced stage and a high degree of nuclear atypia in these tumours. Prognosis appears better for women under 40 years of age.

They considered further therapy could be witheld if tumours were small (5 cm or less in diameter) showing no sign of rupture, and where the histological picture is not too grave. They also thought the contralateral ovary may be saved in women fitting these criteria who wished for future fertility. Evans et al. (1980) estimate the risk of dying from stage Ia(i) granulosa cell tumour in a young woman as 7.5% and only 8.9% risk of developing a recurrence. However, they do point out that in the event of a recurrence the tumour is lethal in 75% of cases and recommended total hysterectomy and bilateral salpingo-oophorectomy after childbearing has finished and total hysterectomy and bilateral salpingo-oophorectomy for any woman with higher stage disease, regardless of reproductive status. They cautioned that one third of recurrences in patients of childbearing age treated by unilateral salpingo-oophorectomy had recurrences in the reproductive tract which would have been removed by initial total hysterectomy and bilateral salpino-oophrectomy. They also considered that radical hysterectomy and pelvic node dissection as unwarranted.

Preoperative or postoperative radiation therapy is advocated by some authors with little data to support this. Evans et al. (1980) found radiation therapy 'of little value'. Stenwig et al. (1979) studied 118 cases with long term follow up, and found that radiotherapy given to patients with early stage disease did not improve the prognosis. 21% recurred as late as 22 years after initial disease. Nearly all authors comment on the value of operative resection of recurrences if they occur, in view of the lack of invasion and aggression shown by all the tumours.

The management of recurrences by chemotherapy has proved difficult. Adjuvant chemotherapy following adequate initial surgical excision is currently being evaluated.

Lusch et al. (1978) reported that a patient aged 58 with a stage Ia tumour developed a recurrence 18 years later. She declined radiotherapy and was treated with melphalan monthly. Her recurrent masses disappeared and she entered a 19 month complete remission.

Malkasian et al. (1974) obtained 3 responses in 12 patients using cyclophosphamide after radiotherapy. Another patient responded to actinomycin D while one treated with melphalan and three treated with 5-fluorouracil showed no response.

Burns et al. (1967) produced one response out of five patients treated with melphalan and Smith and Rutledge (1970) reported six partial responses amongst

15 patients using various alkylating agents, mainly melphalan.

Di Saia et al. (1978) reported a case of recurrent granulosa cell tumour of the ovary that had failed irradiation therapy and alkylating agent plus antimetabolite chemotherapy, and then entered a complete but temporary response following the administration of adriamycin. Barlow et al. (1973) induced a complete response in a patient with a combination of adriamycin and bleomycin but survival was only 11 months.

Live brucellosis vaccine, *Brucella abortus*, administered intraperitoneally, intravenously, subcutaneously or into a tumorous nodule, according to Litvinkova et al. (1980) inhibits the growth of granulosa cell ovarian tumour. However, they found that pretreatment with *Brucella abortus* led, in some experiments, to causing stimulation of tumour growth.

Schwartz and Smith (1976) found that survival after recurrence of granulosa cell tumours was related to the extent of the residual disease after surgery for the recurrence. They treated nine patients with melphalan and none had a complete response and only one a partial lasting for only 7 months. Four patients were given triethylene thiophosphoramide producing one partial response. A combination of actinomycin D, 5-fluorouracil and cyclophosphamide produced two dramatic and prolonged complete responses. They also mention two patients with Sertoli-Leydig tumours who were treated with vincristine, actinomycin D and cyclophosphamide and were both free of disease at the time of reporting despite considerable volumes of recurrent tumour. Another patient with a Sertoli-Leydig cell tumour was given methotrexate along with radiotherapy and died 32 months after the recurrence.

Sertoli-Leydig cell tumours of the ovary

The name Sertoli-Leydig cell tumour (androblastoma) is preferred to the original 'arrhenoblastoma' of Meyer which implies masculinisation, and although most of these tumours do cause such effects, some are endocrinologically quiescent.

According to Scully (1977) they are about 20% as common as granulosa cell tumours, ie less than 0.5% of all ovarian tumours. Roth et al. (1981) reported only one death due to tumour out of 34 cases. The patient had a poorly differentiated tumour and the authors concluded that the better-differentiated tumours have a relatively favourable prognosis. They quoted mortality rates in other series of 3% and 34% and a recurrence/metastasis rate of between 12 and 22% reported in the literature. The patient who died in the Roth et al. series had an abdominal recurrence and elevated androgen levels 16 months after initial surgery. Low dose chlorambucil therapy produced pain relief and improvement of her general condition. One month later her abdomen became more distended and she was commenced on treosulphan lg/day producing a transient reduction in tumour size.

References

Barlow, J. J., Piver, M. S., Chuang, J. T., Cortes, E. P., Ohnuma, T., Holland, J. F., Adriamycin and bleomycin alone and in combination in gynecologic cancers. *Cancer*, 1973, **32**, 735–43.

Björkholm, E., Patterson, F., Granulosa cell and theca cell tumours. The clinical picture and long term outcome for Radiumhemmet series. *Acta Obstet. Gynecol. Scand.*, 1980, **58(4)**, 361–5.

Björkholm, E., Silfverswärd, C., Granulosa and theca cell tumours: Incidence and occurrence of second primary tumours. *Acta Radiol. Oncol. Radiat. Phys. Biol.*, 1980, **19(3)**, 161–7.

Björkholm, E., Silfverswärd, C., Prognostic factors in granulosa cell tumours. *Gynecologic Oncology*, 1981, **11**, 261–74.

Burns, B. C., Rutledge, F. N., Smith, J. P., Delclos, L., Management of ovarian carcinoma: Surgery, irradiation and chemotherapy. *Am. J. Obstet. Gynecol.*, 1967, **98**, 374–83.

Busby, T., Anderson, G. W., Feminizing mesenchymomas of the ovary: includes 107 cases of granulosa-theca cell, and theca cell tumours. *Am. J. Obstet. Gynecol.*, 1954, **68**, 1391–1420.

Di Saia, P., Saltz, A., Kagan, A. R., Rich, W., A temporary response of recurrent granulosa cell tumour to adriamycin. *Obstet. Gynecol.*, 1978, **52**, 355–8.

Evans, A. T., III, Gaffey, T. A., Malkasian, G. D., Annegers, J. F., Clinicopathologic review of 118 granulosa and 82 theca cell tumours. *Obstet. Gynecol.*, 1980, **55**, 231–8.

Fox, H., Agrawal, K., Langley, F. A., A clinicopathologic study of 92 cases of granulosa cell tumour of ovary with special reference to the factors influencing prognosis. *Cancer*, 1975, **35**, 231–41.

Laczkovics, A., Unusual course and site of metastases of a granulosa cell tumour. *Wein Klin Wochenschr.*, 1977, **80**, 315–19.

Litvinkova, P., Trubcheninova, L. P., Baryshnikov, A. I., Effect of *Brucella abortus* on growth of ovarian granulosa cell carcinoma. *Biull. Eksp. Biol. Med.*, 1980, **90, (ii)**, 600–2.

Lusch, C. J., Mercurio, T. M., Runyon, W. K., Delayed recurrence and chemotherapy of a granulosa cell tumour. *Obstet. Gynecol.*, 1978, **51**, 505–7.

Malkasian, G. D., Jr, Webb, M. J., Jorgenson, E. O., Observation on chemotherapy of granulosa cell carcinoma and malignant ovarian teratomas. *Obstet. Gynecol.*, 1974, **44**, 885–88.

Pankratz, E., Boyes, D. A., White, G. W., Galliford, B. W., Fairey, R. N., Benedet, J. L., Granulosa cell tumours. A clinical review of 61 cases. *Obstet. Gynecol.*, 1978, **52**, 718–23.

Roth, L. M., Anderson, M. C., Govan, A. D. T., Langley, F. A., Gowing, N. F. C., Woodcock, A. S., Sertoli-Leydig cell tumours. *Cancer*, 1981, **48**, 187–97.

Schwartz, P. E., Smith, J. P., Treatment of ovarian stromal tumours. *Am. J. Obstet. Gynecol.*, 1976, **125**, 402–11.

Scully, R. E., Sex cord stromal tumours. In Blaustein, A., ed., *Pathology of the female genital tract*. Heidelberg, Springer Verlag, 1977, 505–26.

Smith, J. P., Rutledge, F. N., Chemotherapy in the treatment of cancer of the ovary. *Am. J. Obstet. Gynecol.*, 1970, **107**, 691–703.

Stenwig, J. T., Hazekemp, J. T., Beecham, J. B., Granulosa cell tumour of ovary: A clinicopathological study of 118 cases with long term follow up. *Gynecol. Oncol.*, 1979, **7**, 136–52.

Chapter Twelve

Dysgerminoma, Malignant Teratoma and Mixed Mesodermal Tumours of Ovary

Dysgerminoma

This tumour, which usually affects young women, was described by Clenot in 1911 and called dysgerminoma by Myer in 1931 (Myer 1931) and represents 2% of all ovarian malignancies. Krepart (1981) in Winnipeg, Canada, recommends conservative surgery for stage Ia lesions of less than 10 cm in young patients wishing to preserve their fertility, provided that there is no ascites and the tumour is a well differentiated pure dysgerminoma. Other more advanced stages need careful management. Lymphatic involvement is common—33% of patients had abnormal lymphangiograms in a series recorded by Markovits et al. (1977). Santesson (1947) reported that 21% of patients had mixed cell types, and other authors report in association with other ovarian tumours and generally poorer prognosis.

Most cases are usually treated successfully by surgery and radiotherapy. Boyes et al. (1978), in Vancouver, reported 25 cases only two of whom died of their disease. Four stage I tumours were found in pregnancy, seven patients had metastases and 46% of patients had tumour spread at the time of initial laparotomy. One patient had a gonadoblastoma in the contralateral ovary. Two patients who developed metastases after several years had complete remission after treatment with cyclophosphamide and have continuing tumour free survivals of 12 and 7 years at the time of reporting. Smith and Rutledge (1970) treated 7 cases with melphalan and did not induce a response in any patient.

Of 15 girls aged 8 to 19 years with malignant ovarian tumours between 1961 and 1975 reported by Jereb et al. (1977) the histologies were as follows: 5 epithelial, 5 dysgerminomas, 4 immature teratomas, 1 granulosa cell tumour. Of 3 patients with stage III dysgerminoma two survived.

Reports of survivals have varied considerably. Pedowitz et al. (1955) reported only a 27% 5 year survival rate in a review of 102 cases. Asadourian and Taylor (1969) reported a 90% 5 year survival rate in a review of 105 cases. Malkasian and Symonds (1964) found a 5 year 50% recurrence rate in conservatively treated cases but that treatment for failure produced an 82% 5 year survival. Bush (1979) reported survival of only one patient out of four with stage III disease and another series of only 6 survivors out of 13 patients with stage III and IV disease.

Despite adequate surgery and radiotherapy treatment failures may still occur and this would suggest a role for chemotherapy. Bush (1979) treated only 2 patients with chemotherapy late in their disease and obtained a good partial remission for eight months with intermittent cyclophosphamide. Krepart (1981) obtained remissions using cyclophosphamide and combination chemotherapy consisting of actinomycin D, 5-fluorouracil, cyclophosphamide, bleomycin and vinblastine.

Cohen and Goldsmith (1977) record several reports that dysgerminoma, like its male counterpart, seminoma, is considered sensitive to radiotherapy and alkylating agents but reported a 17 year old patient with progressive, widespread disease despite radiotherapy, alkylating agent and actinomycin D therapy. In view of the patient's leukopoenia the choice of further chemotherapy was limited. They chose vincristine and high dose bleomycin therapy which caused the patient to enter into a complete remission, and followed with vincristine and methotrexate maintenance therapy to avoid pulmonary toxicity associated with high dose bleomycin treatment. Therapy was discontinued after 2 years and they were able to report a 4 year complete chemotherapeutic remission and possible cure. They and several other authors since draw the obvious extrapolation of the successful treatment of germ cell tumours in young men using cisplatin, vinblastine and bleomycin to possible benefits in the treatment of dysgerminoma in young women.

Malignant teratoma

Malignant teratomas of ovary are rare and represent only 0.6% of all ovarian malignancies but as much as 25% of all ovarian malignancies affecting girls. They are nearly always unilateral (Wisniewski and Deppisch 1973).

Curry et al. (1978) reported that prior to the use of combination chemotherapy the prognosis was poor irrespective of stage or grade of tumour. They confirmed that neither postoperative irradiation nor single agent chemotherapy eg methotrexate, 5-fluorouracil or vincristine, was beneficial.

However, two combinations—MAC (methotrexate, actinomycin D and cyclophosphamide) and ActFuCy (actinomycin D, 5-fluorouracil and cyclophosphamide) produced encouraging results. They then progressed to VAC (vincristine, actinomycin D, cyclophosphamide) and have treated 9 patients with advanced stage and 3 patients with early stage disease. Of these, two patients died of their disease 3 and 26 months after chemotherapy had commenced, and the remainder were surviving; of these 6 were in complete continuing remission (16 to 68 months) confirmed by second look laparotomy.

Cangir et al. (1978) treated 8 patients with malignant teratomas of varying stages using vincristine, actinomycin D and cyclophosphamide at M. D. Anderson Hospital and Tumor Institute, Houston, Texas, and all were alive without evidence of disease between 24+ and 80+ months at the time of reporting.

Mixed mesodermal tumour

The chemotherapy of mixed mesodermal tumour of the ovary was discussed fully by Lele et al. (1980) and a report made on 35 cases, 1960–79, at Roswell Park Memorial Institute, Buffalo, New York. Virchow in 1864 coined the term 'carcinosarcoma' but when the sarcomatous elements contain heterologous tissue the term mixed mesodermal tumour is used. A homologous tumour contains sarcoma arising from normal ovarian tissue but in the heterologous tumours the sarcomatous elements are non-ovarian, for example muscle, cartilage and bone. Only 5 cases of Lele et al. (1980) were heterologous.

Twenty four patients received single or multiple agent first line chemotherapy, producing an overall response rate of only 12%. Complete responses were obtained with VAC and with actinomycin D, 5-fluorouracil and cyclophosphamide. A partial remission was obtained with methotrexate, adriamycin and cyclophosphamide. A partial response was obtained with VAC, and second and third line chemotherapy using cisplatin and DTIC produced another partial response. Other varied combinations were unsuccessful. Lele et al. were unsure of why ovarian sarcomas respond so infrequently compared with other sarcomas.

References

Asadourian, L. E., Taylor, H., Dysgerminoma—an analysis of 105 cases. *Obstet. Gynecol.*, 1969, **33**, 370–9.

Boyes, D. A., Pankratz, E., Galliford, B. W., White, G. W., Fairey, R. N., Experience with dysgerminoma at the Cancer Control Agency of British Columbia. *Gynecologic Oncology*, 1978, **6**, 123–9.

Bush, R. S., *Malignancies of the ovary, uterus and cervix*. Edward Arnold, 1979, p. 93.

Cangir, A., Smith, J., van Eys, J., Improved prognosis in children with ovarian cancers following modified VAC (vincristine sulfate, dactinomycin and cyclophosphamide therapy) chemotherapy. *Cancer*, 1978, **42**, 1234–8.

Cohen, S. M., Goldsmith, M. A., Prolonged chemotherapeutic remission of metastatic ovarian dysgerminoma. Report of a case. *Gynecologic Oncology*, 1977, **5**, 299–304.

Curry, S. L., Smith, J. P., Gallagher, H. S., Malignant teratoma of the ovary—prognostic factors and treatment. *Am. J. Obstet. Gynecol.*, 1978, **131**, 845.

Jereb, B., Golouh, R., Havlicek, S., Ovarian cancer in children and adolescents: a review of 15 cases. *Med. Pediatr. Oncol.*, 1977, **3(4)**, 339–43.

Krepart, G. V., The treatment of ovarian dysgerminoma. In *Gynecologic Oncology— Controversies in Cancer Treatment*. ed. Ballon, S. C., G. K. Hall & Co., 1981, p. 356–61.

Lele, S. B., Piver, S., Barlow, J. J., Chemotherapy in the management of mixed mesodermal tumours of the ovary. *Gynecologic Oncology*, 1980, **10**, 298–302.

Malkasian, G. D., Symonds, R. E., Treatment of the unilateral encapsulated ovarian dysgerminoma. *Amer. J. Obstet. Gynecol.*, 1964, **90**, 379–82.

Markovits, P., Bergiron, C., Chauvel, C., Castellino, R. A., Lymphography in the staging, treatment planning and surveillance of ovarian dysgerminomas. *Am. J. Roentgenol.*, 1977, **128**, 835–8.

Myer, R., The pathology of some special ovarian tumours and their relationship to sex characteristics. *Am. J. Obstet. Gynecol.*, 1931, **22**, 697–710.

Pedowitz, P., Felmus, L. B., Grayzel, D. M., Dysgerminoma of ovary: prognosis and treatment. *Am. J. Obstet. Gynecol.*, 1955, **70**, 1284–97.

Santesson, L., Clinical and pathological survey of ovarian tumours treated at Radium-hemmet. 1: dysgerminoma. *Acta Radiol. (Stockholm)*, 1947, **28**, 644–68.

Smith, J. P., Rutledge, F., Chemotherapy for carcinoma of the ovary. *Am. J. Obstet. Gynecol.*, 1970, **107**, 691–700.

Wisniewski, M., Deppisch, L. M., Solid teratomas of the ovary. *Cancer*, 1973, **32**, 440.

Chapter Thirteen

Endodermal Sinus Tumours of Ovary

Teilum recognised in 1946 the resemblance of Schiller's mesonephromas of ovary (1939) to the yolk sac endoderm of the rat placenta and renamed them endodermal sinus tumours, more in keeping with its extraembryonal germ cell origin; and later in 1974 found that alpha feto-protein is synthesised by cells of the yolk sac endoderm lining the endodermal sinuses.

It is a highly malignant and uncommon tumour of the ovary (and other extragonadal sites) occurring mainly in children and young adults. Forney et al. (1975) discussed 102 cases and all but 10 of these were dead within two years of diagnosis, and all of the survivors had stage Ia tumours. Kurman and Norris (1976a) reported on 65 cases; the three-year survival rate was only 13%. Jimmerson and Woodruff (1977) reported on 34 cases, only three of which had survived. Moreover, Kurman and Norris (1976b) pointed out that mixed germ cell tumours containing more than 33% of endodermal sinus tumour elements and measuring more than 10 cm in diameter proved invariably to be fatal.

Most of these patients were treated by surgery alone or in combination with radiotherapy but Gallion et al. (1979) concluded that neither radiotherapy nor removal of the uterus and contralateral ovary improved the survival of patients with this tumour.

However, evidence is gradually accumulating to support the suggestion that the addition of chemotherapy to conservative surgery may improve survivals considerably (Karlen and Kastelic 1980).

Table 13.1 gives a summary of the reported experience of treating endodermal sinus tumours of ovary with chemotherapy.

Extragonadal endodermal sinus tumours are very uncommon and have been reported in the pelvis, vagina, sacrococcygeal region, mediastinum, liver, retroperitoneum and central nervous system by Thomas et al. (1981) who also successfully treated two patients who had failed on VAC (vincristine, actinomycin D, cyclophosphamide) with cisplatin, vinblastine, adriamycin and bleomycin.

Serum alpha feto-protein, the normal alpha-globulin of human fetal serum first described by Bergstrand and Czar (1956), has proved useful as a tumour marker in the management of patients with endodermal sinus tumours or mixed germ cell tumours of the ovary containing endodermal sinus tumour elements whose serum alpha fetoprotein is raised before initiating chemotherapy. A fall in alpha feto-

Table 13.1   Chemotherapy of endodermal sinus tumours

Agent(s)/Source	No. of patients	No. responding	Continuing survival (months)
Vincristine			
Actinomycin D			
Cyclophosphamide			
Jimmerson (1977)	1	1	25
Smith (1975)	20	14	3–78
Williamson (1973)	1	0	—
Danforth (1978)	1	1	37
Slayton (1978)	16	9	14–55
Ungerleider (1978)	4	3	26–51
Weed (1979)	1	0	— (recurrence during pregnancy)
Cangir (1978)	6	4	32–79
	6 (mixed germ cell tumours)	3	18–120
Gallion (1979)	1	1	24
Karlen (1980)	1	1	39 (subsequent successful pregnancy)
Kurman (1976)	4	3	>24
VAC ±			
Adriamycin			
Cisplatin			
Bleomycin			
Etoposide			
Romero (1981)	4	3	10–36
	2 (mixed germ cell tumours)	1	60
Actinomycin D			
5-Fluorouracil			
Cyclophosphamide			
Karlen (1980)	1	1	36
Forney (1975)	2	2	27, 33
Smith (1975)	8	1	57
Slayton (1978)	1	0	—
Methotrexate			
Actinomycin D			
Chlorambucil			
Creasman (1979)	5	3	3–48
Duncan (1980)	1	1	48 (subsequent successful pregnancy)
Huntingdon (1970)	1	0	—
Bleomycin			
Vinblastine			
Actinomycin D			
Methotrexate			
Sell (1976)	6	2	8–11

protein to less than 20 ng/ml followed by any subsequent elevation is suggestive of recurrent or progressive disease (Romero and Schwartz 1981). However, the same authors at the Yale University School of Medicine caution that a negative alpha fetoprotein level in the blood does not eliminate the possibility of recurrent disease and that patients should be assessed clinically. They also recommend serial alpha feto-protein measurements on a monthly basis using radio-immunoassay and not other less sensitive techniques—see also *Assessment of response* in Chapter 4.

Duncan and Young (1980) in Dundee, Scotland, reported a successful pregnancy after unilateral oophorectomy and adjuvant chemotherapy. The levels of serum alpha feto-protein were within the normal range during the pregnancy and undetectable before and afterwards.

References

Bergstrand, C., Czar, B., Demonstration of a new protein fraction in serum of human fetus. *Scand. J. Clin. Lab. Invest.*, 1956, **8**, 174–8.

Cangir, A., Smith, J., van Eys, J., Improved prognosis in children with ovarian cancers following modified VAC (vincristine, dactinomycin and cyclophosphamide) chemotherapy. *Cancer*, 1978, **42**, 1234–8.

Creasman, W. T., Felter, B. F., Hammond, C. B., Parker, R. T., Germ cell malignancies of the ovary. *Obstet. Gynecol.*, 1979, **53**, 226.

Danforth, D. N., Dird, C. C., Victor, T. A., Endodermal sinus tumour of the ovary: the orphan tumour. *Obstet. Gynecol.*, 1978, **51**, 233.

Duncan, I. D., Young, J. L., Endodermal sinus tumours of the ovary: serum alpha feto-protein levels before and after treatment and during pregnancy. *Br. J. Obstet. Gynae.*, 1980, **87**, 535–8.

Forney, J. P., DiSaia, P. J., Morrow, C. P., Endodermal sinus tumour: A report of two sustained remissions treated with a combination of actinomycin D, 5-fluorouracil and cyclophosphamide. *Obstet. Gynecol.*, 1975, **45**, 186.

Gallion, H., van Nagell, J. R., Powell, D. F., Donaldson, E. S., Hanson, M., Therapy of endodermal sinus tumours of the ovary. *Am. J. Obstet. Gynecol.*, 1979, **135**, 447.

Huntingdon, R. W., Bullock, W. K., Yolk sac tumors of the ovary. *Cancer*, 1970, **25**, 1357–67.

Jimmerson, G. K., Woodruff, J. D., Ovarian extraembryonal teratomas: 1. endodermal sinus tumor. *Am. J. Obstet. Gynecol.*, 1977, **127**, 73.

Karlen, J. R., Kastelic, J. E., Endodermal sinus tumor of the ovary: an improving prognosis. *Gynecologic Oncology*, 1980, **10**, 206–16.

Kurman, R. J., Norris, H. J., Endodermal sinus tumor of the ovary: a clinical and pathologic analysis of 71 cases. *Cancer*, 1976a, **38**, 2404–19.

Kurman, R. J., Norris, H. J., Malignant mixed germ cell tumor of the ovary. A clinical and pathologic analysis of 30 cases. *Obstet. Gynecol.*, 1976b, **48**, 579.

Romero, R., Schwartz, P. E., Alpha-fetoprotein determination in the management of endodermal sinus tumor and mixed germ cell tumor of the ovary. *Am. J. Obstet. Gynecol.*, 1981, **141**, 126–31.

Schiller, W., Mesonephroma ovarii. *Am. J. Cancer*, 1939, **35**, 1–21.

Sell, A., Sogaard, H., Norgaard-Pedersen, B., Serum alpha fetoprotein as a marker for the effect of postoperative radiation therapy and/or chemotherapy in eight cases of ovarian endodermal sinus tumour. *Int. J. Cancer*, 1976, **18**, 574–80.

Slayton, R. E., Hreshchyshyn, M. D., Silverberg, C. G., Treatment of malignant ovarian germ cell tumors: response to vincristine, dactinomycin and cyclophosphamide (preliminary report). *Cancer*, 1978, **42**, 390.

Smith, J. P., Rutledge, F., Advances in the chemotherapy for gynecologic cancer. *Cancer*, 1975, **36** (Suppl.), 669.

Teilum, G., Gonocytoma: homolous ovarian and testicular tumours 1. with discussion of 'mesonephroma ovarii' (Schiller, *Am. J. Cancer*, 1939). *Acta Pathol. Microbiol. Scand.*, 1946, **23**, 242–51.

Teilum, G., Albrechtsen, R., Norgaard-Pedersen, B., Immunofluorescent localisation of alpha fetoprotein synthesis in endodermal sinus tumour (yolk sac tumour). *Acta Pathol. Microbiol. Scand.* (A), 1974, **82**, 586–8.

Thomas, W. J., Kelleher, J. F., Duval-Arnould, B., Successful treatment of metastatic extragonadal endodermal sinus (yolk sac) tumor in childhood. *Cancer*, 1981, **48**, 2371–4.

Ungerlieder, R. S., Donaldson, S. S., Warnke, R. A., Wilbur, J. R., Endodermal sinus tumour: The Stanford experience and the first reported case arising in the vulva. *Cancer*, 1978, **41**, 1627.

Weed, J. C., Roh, R. A., Mendenhall, H. W., Recurrent endodermal sinus tumor during pregnancy. *Obstet. Gynecol.*, 1979, **54**, 653.

Chapter Fourteen

Gestational Trophoblastic Tumours

Although trophoblastic neoplasms are uncommon, choriocarcinoma occurs in 1 in 40 000 pregnancies in England and Wales (Bagshawe 1969), they illustrate fundamental principles concerning the chemotherapy of solid tumours in general and the national and international cooperation required for the investigation and management of rare tumours. Before the introduction of chemotherapy, the mortality of choriocarcinoma was high—Ober et al. (1971) estimated a survival rate of only 19%.

Centralised management

If patients with uncommon tumours are managed by a few centres covering large areas much more experience in the treatment of these conditions will be obtained than if the patients are dealt with by local practitioners who see the condition infrequently. Data on these tumours, their incidence, chemosensitivity, pathology and so forth, may be accumulated quickly, centralised and computerised. Patterns of resistance may be identified along with prognostic factors so that therapeutic strategy may be modified relatively speedily.

Such systems in the world do operate for trophoblastic disease and data on this uncommon tumour are readily available. In the United Kingdom patients are registered with the Royal College of Obstetricians and Gynaecologists and their management directed by Charing Cross Hospital, London, or Sheffield, or Dundee in Scotland. Lewis (1980) in his Presidential Address to the New York Obstetrical Society acknowledges that 'no centre has made more important contributions to our understanding and treatment of gestational choriocarcinoma than the unit at Charing Cross Hospital, London, England, under the direction of Prof Kenneth Bagshawe.' This is in contradistinction to the management of some common tumours, eg of the breast and ovary, where lack of standardisation of treatment via centralised control centres with rapid data retrieval systems has prejudiced treatment progress.

In view of the excellent chances of successful treatment patients should be referred to these special centres in the UK and USA, and practitioners without such experience and expertise should not be tempted to treat these patients independently.

Tumour markers

Trophoblastic disease offers an excellent model to illustrate the use of a tumour marker for diagnosis, the detection of residual and/or recurrent disease and for monitoring chemotherapy. Treated patients requiring follow-up can submit to the central controlling unit urine with or without serum for analysis and obviate the need for attendance at time-consuming outpatient clinics. Human chorionic gonadotrophin (HCG) is currently employed as the marker of choice in this condition but others have been put forward (see Chapter 5, page 30).

Cure rates

The majority of even the most highly malignant forms of trophoblastic cancer are now cured using chemotherapy without the use of radiotherapy and extensive surgery. Adjunctive radiotherapy is occasionally used for advanced disease. Li and Hertz (1956) cured the first patient with metastatic gestational trophoblastic cancer using only one cytotoxic agent, ie methotrexate. This was hoped to open the way for many other solid tumour cures to be obtained solely by the use of cytotoxic agents, a hope which, despite the increasingly successful treatment of choriocarcinoma, testicular teratoma and other unusual tumours, has remained largely unfulfilled. However, by 1965 75% of patients were being cured (5 year disease free survival) using methotrexate and/or actinomycin D (Ross et al. 1965) while Bagshawe and McDonald (1960) added 6-mercaptopurine to the methotrexate, as compared to only about 25% using methotrexate alone (Bagshawe 1977).

Further combinations were then introduced so that by 1978 the reported cure rate was 90% (Lewis 1980) and 100% for low risk patients treated in referral centres using single agents and reserving combination chemotherapy for poor responders and high risk patients.

A popular combination in the USA was an alkylating agent, methotrexate and actinomycin D (Surwit et al. 1979) whereas Bagshawe (1977) introduced CHAMOMA, ie hydroxyurea, vincristine, methotrexate, actinomycin D, cyclophosphamide, adriamycin and melphalan (see later) which successfully treated cases resistant to earlier triple therapy.

Hydatidiform mole

After diagnosis and evacuation the patient should be observed with serial HCG assays at a referral centre. In about 90% of patients further treatment is unnecessary. Bagshawe et al. (1973) recommend chemotherapy in those patients whose urinary HCG levels remain above 40 000 iu per 24 hours at 4–6 weeks post evacuation, or any raised HCG levels 5–6 months post-evacuation. Of course, evidence of metastases is also an indication for chemotherapy.

In the USA the criteria of Goldstein and Berkowitz (1980) or Hammond et al. (1973) have been adopted and current practice is to diagnose nonmetastatic trophoblastic disease on the basis of three plateau values of HCG over a period of two weeks ie days X, X + 7, and X + 14 (Kohorn 1982) and this leads to a higher chemotherapy rate ie 26%. Kohorn (1982) presents data to suggest that a plateau of three or four weeks may be justified, more in keeping with the Bagshawe (1976) criteria.

Prognostic factors

High cure rates have been obtained by dividing patients into risk groups, reserving combination chemotherapy for the medium and high risk groups.

Hammond et al. (1973) reported a 70% complete remission rate in high risk patients treated initially with combination chemotherapy compared with only

Table 14.1   Prognostic scoring for trophoblastic tumours (from Bagshawe, 1977)

Risk factor	Score = 0	10	20	40
Age (yr)	<39	>39		
Parity	1, 2, >4	3 or 4		
Antecedent pregnancy	Mole	Abortion	Term	
Interval (antecedent pregnancy—chemotherapy) in months	<3	4–7	7–12	>12
hCG (plasma mIU/ml or urine IU/day)	10^3–10^4	$<10^3$	10^4–10^5	$>10^5$
ABO groups (patient and husband)	A × A × B × AB	O × O A × O	B × AB ×	
No. of metastases	—	1–4	4–8	>8
Site of metastases	Not detected Lungs Vagina	Spleen Kidney	Gastrointestinal tract Liver	Brain
Largest tumor mass (cm)	<3	3–5	>5	
Lymphocytic infiltration	Marked	Moderate, unknown	Slight	
Immune status	Reactive		Unreactive	
Previous chemotherapy	—		Yes	

14% in similar patients when combination chemotherapy was given after the failure of single agent therapy. Low risk patients should expect 100% complete remission rates (Jones and Lewis 1974).

A prognostic score based upon a variety of factors was prepared by Bagshawe (1976)—see Table 14.1

Bagshawe et al. (1971) reported that ABO blood group differences between the patient and her husband influences prognosis. Lawler (1978) showed that patients with hydatidiform moles have a high chance of developing antibodies to paternal HLA antigens, and that the complete mole is derived from an XX zygote with only a duplicated male haplotype with no female contribution of X chromosomes (Lawler et al. 1979).

The total prognostic score is calculated: low risk <60, medium risk 60–90 and high risk >90. Bagshawe (1978) reported that out of 64 patients with chorio-carcinoma who died, 45 succumbed to drug resistance.

Patients taking the oral contraceptive pill following a hydatidiform mole may demonstrate delay in the disappearance of the trophoblast, occasionally requiring chemotherapy (Stone et al. 1976).

Treatment

A variety of single agents show activity in gestational choriocarcinoma.

Low risk

In recent years the Charing Cross Hospital team has treated low risk patients with a prognostic score of less than 60 using methotrexate and folinic acid rescue alone, with small doses given frequently until the HCG level falls (Bagshawe 1977a). Should methotrexate fail to eliminate HCG an alternative therapy with vin-cristine, actinomycin D and cyclophosphamide may be chosen. Chemotherapy is continued for approximately two to three months after the HCG is no longer detectable since HCG assays are not sensitive enough to detect the production from less than 10^4–10^5 tumour cells (Bagshawe 1977).

Medium risk

To avoid resistance in the medium risk 60–90 score group a sequential form of therapy is recommended consisting of actinomycin D, vincristine, cyclo-phosphamide, hydroxyurea, methotrexate, folinic acid and 6-mercaptopurine (Bagshawe 1977a). Recently induction with VP16-213 (etoposide) has been added to that regimen: 100 mg/m^2 in 200 ml of saline, intravenously for five consecutive days.

High risk

High risk in excess of 90 score patients have been treated with CHAMOMA, ie the regimen for medium risk patients with the addition of adriamycin and melphalan. Surwit et al. (1979) modified this Bagshawe high risk regimen by adding additional actinomycin D and produced complete remissions in five out of six patients who had developed resistance to MAC (methotrexate, actinomycin D and cyclophosphamide) therapy. Jones (1981) modified CHAMOMA using the same agents in a different sequence with additional vincristine. Of eight resistant patients all showed an initial response, one obtained a complete remission and two patients were alive with disease. Recently Charing Cross Hospital have been using CHAMOCA omitting melphalan in a nine day course with relatively few side effects and myelosuppression which usually recovers after two weeks.

Drug resistant patients have also been successfully treated using additional agents such as VP16-213 (etoposide) and cisplatinum (Newlands and Bagshawe

1980, Lurain and Piver 1980). Vindesine (desacetyl vinblastine amide sulphate), the vinca alkaloid analogue, has also been evaluated (Currie et al. 1978).

Results

Approximately 20% of low risk patients and 40% of medium and high risk patients will develop drug resistance requiring a change of treatment. Between 1974 and 1979 only one patient out of 70 in the low risk group died of chorio-carcinoma at the Charing Cross Hospital, only one out of 38 in the medium risk group, and only seven out of 41 in the high risk group.

It has become apparent that about 90% of patients with this rare and lethal cancer, managed by an experienced referral centre using accurate tumour marker assays and effective chemotherapy, can be offered a cure. This exciting example of tumour diagnosis, follow up and treatment with chemotherapy alone cannot fail to stimulate all to seek the same level of control in other solid tumours.

References

Bagshawe, K. D., McDonald, J. M., Treatment of choriocarcinoma with a combination of cytotoxic drugs. *Br. Med. J.*, 1960, **2**, 426.

Bagshawe, K. D., In *Choriocarcinoma: the clinical aspects and biology of the trophoblast and its tumours*. Edward Arnold, 1969, London.

Bagshawe, K. D., Rawlins, G., Pike, M. C., Lawler, S. D., ABO blood-groups in trophoblastic neoplasia. *Lancet*, 1971, **1**, 553–7.

Bagshawe, K. D., Wilson, H., Dublon, P., Smith, A., Baldwin, M., Kardana, A., Follow up after hydatidiform mole: studies using radioimmunoassay for urinary human chorionic gonadotrophin (HCG). *J. Obstet. Gynecol Brit. Commwth.*, 1973, **80**, 461–8.

Bagshawe, K. D., Risk and prognostic factors in trophoblastic neoplasia. *Cancer*, 1976, **38**, 1373.

Bagshawe, K. D., Treatment of trophoblastic tumours. *Recent Results Cancer Res.*, 1977a, **62**, 192.

Bagshawe, K. D., Presidential Address: lessons from choriocarcinoma. *Proc. Roy. Soc. Med.*, 1977, **70**, 303–6.

Bagshawe, K. D., Trophoblastic disease. ed. Caplan R. M., Sweeney, W. J. III, in *Advances in Obstetrics and Gynecology*, 1978, Baltimore, Williams & Wilkins Co., 225–37.

Currie, V. E., Wong, P., Krakoff, I. H., Young, C. W., Phase I trial of vindesine in patients with advanced cancer. *Cancer Treat. Rep.*, 1978, **62**, 1333–6.

Goldstein, D. P., Berkowitz, R. S., Management of gestational trophoblastic neoplasms. *Curr. Probl. Obstet. Gynecol.*, 1980, **3**, 5.

Hammond, C. B., Borchert, L. G., Tyrey, L., Creasman, W. T., Parker, R. T., Treatment of metastatic trophoblastic disease: Good and poor prognosis. *Am. J. Obstet. Gynecol.*, 1973, **115**, 451.

Jones, W. B., Lewis, J. L., Jr., Treatment of gestational trophoblastic disease. *Am. J. Obstet. Gynecol.*, 1974, **120**, 14.

Jones, W. B., Trophoblastic tumours—prognostic factors. *Cancer*, 1981, **48**, 602–7.

Kohorn, E. I., Criteria toward the definition of nonmetastatic gestational trophoblastic disease after hydatidiform mole. *Am. J. Obstet. Gynecol.*, 1982, **142**, 416.

Lawler, S. D., HLA and trophoblastic tumours. *Br. Med. Bull.*, 1978, **34**(3), 305–8.

Lawler, S. D., Povey, S., Evans, M. W., Szulman, A. E., Genetic studies of complete and partial hydatidiform moles. *Lancet*, 1979, **2**, 580.

Lewis, J. L., Treatment of metastatic gestational trophoblastic neoplasms. *Am. J. Obstet. Gynec.*, 1980, **136**, 163–72..

Li, M. C., Hertz, R., Spencer, D. B., Effect of methotrexate therapy on choriocarcinoma and chorioadenoma. *Proc. Soc. Biol. Med.*, 1956, **93**, 361.

Lurain, J. R., Piver, M. S., Metastatic gestational trophoblastic disease—secondary chemotherapy. *N. Y. State J. Med.*, 1980, **80**, 234–7.

Newlands, E. S., Bagshawe, K. D., Antitumour activity of the epipodophyllin derivative VP16-213 (Etoposide: NSG-141540) in gestational choriocarcinoma. *Eur. J. Cancer*, 1980, **16**, 401–5.

Ober, W. B., Edgcomb, J. H., Price, E. D., Jr., The pathology of choriocarcinoma. *Ann. N.Y. Acad. Sci.*, 1971, **172**, 299–426.

Ross, G. T., Goldstein, D. P., Hertz, R., Lipsett, M. B., Odell, W. D., Sequential use of methotrexate and actinomycin D in the treatment of metastatic choriocarcinoma and related trophoblastic diseases in women. *Am. J. Obstet. Gynecol.*, 1965, **93**, 223.

Stone, M., Dent, J., Kardana, A., Bagshawe, K. D., Relationship of oral contraception to development of trophoblastic tumour after evacuation of a hydatidiform mole. *Br. J. Obstet. Gynae.*, 1976, **83**, 913.

Surwit, E. A., Suciu, T. N., Schmidt, H. J., Hammond, C. B., A new combination chemotherapy for resistant trophoblastic disease. *Gynecologic Oncology*, 1979, **8**, 110–18.

Chapter Fifteen

Carcinoma of the Cervix

The role of chemotherapy in the treatment of cancer of the cervix is not clear.

Some clinicians have relegated its role to that of pain relief and palliation; and many are reluctant to contemplate any interference with standard surgical and radiotherapeutic treatment programmes until effective chemotherapy can be shown to be of clear benefit.

It is true that the management of cervical cancer by surgery and/or radiotherapy, compared to that of most other solid tumours, is, indeed, a success story and that very serious thought should be given to any schedules planning to include the introduction of chemotherapy, either as primary treatment, or upon an adjuvant basis.

However, two facts have become clear: firstly, all attempts to treat recurrent carcinoma of the cervix using chemotherapy have been largely unsuccessful—see Tables 15.1 and 15.2; secondly, half of the patients with this tumour will eventually die of their disease, and this modifies, in real terms, the description of successful in regard to current surgery and radiotherapeutic management.

These surgical and radiotherapeutic principles have not changed significantly over the last 50 years, although there have been alterations in techniques. Mortality rates in the UK and USA have gradually fallen (Hill 1975) with now just over 2000 deaths per annum in England and Wales, and approximately 8000 in the USA (Wasserman and Carter 1977). Among those who die of this tumour are young and middle aged women with large family commitments whose untimely death inflicts considerable social trauma. Of 318 patients with progressive disease treated with chemotherapy at the Mayo Clinic, the mean age was 49 years and the range 15 to 74 years (Malkasian 1977).

Some would suggest that improvement in overall results in this disease is not necessarily due to improvement in radiotherapeutic techniques but by screening methods detecting lesions in the earlier stages (Jolles 1980). Even in those centres where results appear best, at least 40% of patients will die of their disease after receiving current surgical and/or radiotherapeutic measures (Bush 1979, Wasserman and Carter 1977)—clearly there is still considerable room for improvement.

Survival after surgery and/or radiotherapy

According to Kottmeier (1976) the five year survival rates of patients with cervical carcinoma are:

Stage I—80%
Stage II—59%   Overall—55%
Stage III—32%
Stage IV—7%

Lederman (1964) reported that the five-year survival rates for all stages in four centres in the UK (1945–54) lay between 40 and 41.3%, in seven centres under 38% and, in one, only 26.1%. Blaikley et al (1962) reported the results of the Royal Marsden and Chelsea Hospitals, London, for the years 1933–60:

Stage I—64%
Stage II—45%
Stage III—19%
Stage IV—4%

Mould and Staffurth (1979) reported the figures for the Royal Marsden, Chelsea, Hammersmith, University College and Middlesex Hospitals, London, 1944–72:

Stage I—71%
Stage II—48%
Stage III—21%

Jolles (1980) reported the long term results of treatment in Northampton, England, of 536 patients treated with radiotherapy alone combined with 66 patients treated by radiotherapy preceding or following hysterectomy:

	1949–53	1964–68	1944–68
Stage I	67%	70%	69%
Stage II	59%	58%	52%
Stage III	33%	25%	25%
Stage IV	1/16	2/24	7/75

giving a crude survival rate of only 41%.

Treatment of recurrent disease

There are a formidable number of factors which prejudice the successful treatment of recurrent cervical carcinoma by chemotherapy:

(1) Chemotherapy reaches its target tumour via the bloodstream—the blood supply may be severely reduced by previous surgery or fibrosis induced following surgery and/or radiotherapy;

(2) the majority of tumours are of squamous cell origin with few chemotherapeutic agents showing significant efficacy against this type of tumour;

(3) many chemotherapy schedules and doses are compromised by the renal failure with which end stage disease is frequently associated;

(4) bone marrow function is often compromised by previous radiotherapy commonly imposing marked dose limiting restrictions when giving chemotherapy as second line treatment;

(5) the tumours do not appear sensitive to hormone manipulation—see below.

(6) assessment of response is notoriously difficult to measure despite the use of ultrasound and computerised axial tomography. Reliable tumour markers with which to follow responses to therapy are also lacking;

(7) experience is still limited and not many patients are given chemotherapy—even the National Cancer Institute in the USA reported that of 4599 patients between 1965 and 1969 only 11% received drugs as part of their therapy (US Dept of Health, Education and Welfare, 1974);

(8) the results of chemotherapy already presented and their possible influence on survival may be, in addition, difficult to interpret in the knowledge that approximately 5% of patients receiving no treatment for recurrent carcinoma of the cervix are alive at two years from diagnosis (Forney et al. 1975).

Tables 15.1 and 15.2 give a review of the attempts to treat recurrent advanced tumours. Whereas any success is reported only in terms of objective remission, some authors have managed to deduce effects on survival. Guthrie and Way (1978) reported prolonged survival, using adriamycin and methotrexate against advanced disease, amongst those patients whose tumours showed response, ie a median survival of 56 weeks (range 10–118) for patients with partial or complete remissions compared with only 20 weeks (range 7–73) in non-responders.

Many authors comment on the grave limitation on any chemotherapy used in such patients caused by myelosuppression secondary to irradiation—perhaps more supportive measures now available may, to some extent, counteract this effect—for example, bone marrow transplantation (Powles et al. 1980).

Piver et al. (1974) reported that hydroxyurea improved survival—choosing this agent for its alleged synergistic effect with radiation rather than direct chemo-therapeutic effect. Bleomycin is popular for inclusion into treatment protocols again for its synergism with radiation (Jorgensen 1972).

Hormone therapy

Varga and Henriksen (1964) reported on 13 patients who were treated with intramuscular hydroxyprogesterone, none of whom showed any objective remission. Malkasian et al. (1977) treated 9 patients with 5-fluorouracil plus 6,17-dimethyl-6-hydroprogesterone with no objective responses, 8 received cyclophosphamide plus 6,17-dimethyl-6-hydroprogesterone with only one objective response. There is no real evidence that these tumours are sensitive to hormones in a manner which could be exploited therapeutically.

Chemotherapy as primary treatment for advanced disease

While radical radiotherapy does offer some, albeit small, chance of survival for patients with very advanced tumours, few units have been prepared to try chemotherapy as an alternative or additional treatment, and yet patients with disseminated disease may well be the group who will benefit from systemic drug administration. However, opportunities have arisen for advanced disease to be treated with chemotherapy as the only treatment—in some cases with remarkable results. Trussell and Mitford-Barberton then in Kampala, Uganda (1961) were faced by a relatively large number of patients with advanced tumours but at that time there were no radiotherapy facilities in East Africa. In cooperation with the Sloan-Kettering Institute in New York, 14 patients with advanced cervical carcinoma were treated with a pelvic infusion of methotrexate via bilateral cannulation of the internal iliac arteries. All patients showed tumour regression, in three cases Wertheim's hysterectomy was made possible, and in one patient the tumour regressed completely.

In contrast, Morrow et al. (1977) in an effort to prolong increased tissue levels with chemotherapy given as second line treatment, ie bleomycin (which has a short half-life of less than 1 hour) (Ohnuma et al. 1974), treated 20 patients (1971–4) with recurrent disease following irradiation using an intra-arterial pelvic infusion but concluded that the theoretical advantage of this treatment proved to be of no clinical importance when the treatment is given for recurrent tumour ie an objective tumour regression rate of 13% and an overall mean survival of 7 months (range 1–19).

Chemotherapy for early stage disease

The patient with positive para-aortic nodes despite early stage disease has a poor outlook despite treatment with surgery and radiotherapy—50% recurring within 2 years of initial treatment (Guthrie and Way 1978) and this may represent a situation whereby systemic chemotherapy should be evaluated. Indeed, the Gynecologic Oncology Group in the USA intends to introduce cisplatin as an adjuvant to radiotherapy in such patients. The USA Gynecologic Oncology Group and the Southwest Oncology Group are also evaluating two drug combinations of cisplatin plus other agents such as cytoxan, adriamycin, ICRF-159, dianhydrogalacititol and mitomycin C, in comparison with cisplatin alone in a variety of dose schedules (Thigpen 1981).

Conclusion

Tate Thigpen and his team at Jackson, Mississippi, USA, told the American Cancer Society National Conference on Gynecologic Cancer (1980) in Los Angeles (Thigpen et al. 1981) that 'the priorities for clinical research in cervix carcinoma include identification of new active drugs, definition of optimal dose and schedule of highly active agents, stepwise development of combinations of highly active agents with documented superiority over single agent therapy, and evaluation of systemic therapy as an adjuvant in high risk, early stage disease.' He has set us all a formidable task—but one which must be tackled in earnest.

Table 15.1   Single agent chemotherapy for carcinoma of the cervix

Agent	Source	No. of patients	% Objective regression
Nitrogen mustard	Smith (1967)	5	0
Cyclophosphamide	Smith (1967)		
	Solidaro (1967)	124	21
	Roy (1967)		
	Malkasian (1977)	40	17
	Latief (1982)	11	27
Chlorambucil	Moore (1968c)	44	30
	Masterson (1965)		
	Latief (1982)	5	0
Thiotepa	Smith (1967)	6	17
	Latief (1982)	2	0
Melphalan	Smith (1967)	20	20
Treosulphan	Latief (1982)	1	0
Hexamethylmelamine	Malkasian (1977)	4	25
	Stolinsky (1973)	21	38
	Wilson (1969)	15	20
	Latief (1982)	3	0
Cisplatin	Thigpen (1981)	34	38
	Thigpen (1978)	18	44 (11%CR, 33%PR)
	Carlson (1981)	9*	30
	Hall (1981)	22	9
	Latief (1982)	14	0
	Cohen (1978)	11	45
BCNU	Carter (1972)	7	14
CCNU	Wasserman (1974a)	5	20
Methyl-CCNU	Wasserman (1974b)	32	13
Etoposide (VP-16)	Slayton (1979)	30	0
ICRF-159	Conroy (1980)	18	5
Methotrexate	Roy (1967)	19	25
	de Palo (1973)	23	25
	Trussell (1961)	14*	100 (1CR, 14PR)
	Cavins (1978)	37	42
	Latief (1982)	19	36 (2CR, 5PR)
6-Mercaptopurine	Masterton (1965)	10	0
	Moore (1968)	18	6
5-Fluorouracil	Ansfield (1962)	17	25
	Moore (1968a)	15	33
	Malkasian (1968)	80	16
	Malkasian (1977)	208	18
DTIC	Goldsmith (1972)	12	25
Hydroxyurea	Smith (1967)	4	0
Vincristine	Hreshchyshyn (1963)	31	29
	Holland (1973)	13	8
Adriamycin	Barlow (1975)	8	25
	Greenberg (1977)	9	45
	Slavik (1975)	20	15
	de Vita (1976)	28	18
	Wallace (1978)	54	17

Table 15.1—continued

Agent	Source	No. of patients	% Objective regression
Bleomycin	Suzuki (1970)	17	0
	Barlow (1973)	6	0
	Blum (1973)	94	24
	De Palo (1973)	23	13
	De Vita (1976)	172	10
	Morrow (1977)	16*	13
	Latief (1982)	8	12
Mitomycin C	Moore (1968d)	18	22

* Intra-arterial infusion

Table 15.2   Combination chemotherapy for carcinoma of the cervix

Agents	Source	No. of patients	% Objective regression
Methotrexate Vincristine	Hakes (1979)	29	17
Methotrexate Bleomycin	Piel (1973)	8	62 (3CR, 2PR)
	Conroy (1976)	20	60
Methotrexate Cyclophosphamide	Roy (1969)	11	0
	Papavasiliou (1969)	23	10 (3CR, 7PR)
Methotrexate Adriamycin	Haid (1977)	16	12
	Piver (1978)	15	0
	Papavasiliou (1978)	26	29
	Guthrie (1978)	48	63
	Latief (1982)	32	19
Adriamycin Bleomycin	Bond (1976)	20	35
	Greenberg (1977)	11	0
	Barlow (1973)	15	13
	Piver (1978)	16	6
	de Palo (1976)	15	20
Adriamycin Cyclophosphamide	Wallace (1978)	39	18
	Alberts (1978)	10	10
Adriamycin Methyl-CCNU	Day (1978)	31	45
Cyclophosphamide Vincristine	de Palo (1976)	19	10
Bleomycin Mitomycin C	Mujamoto (1978)	15	93 (12CR, 2PR)
	Leichman (1980)	19	16 (1CR, 2PR)
Adriamycin Cisplatin	Slayton (1978)	19	32

Table 15.2—continued

Agent	Source	No. of patients	% Objective regression
Adriamycin *Vincristine* *Methotrexate*	Wallace (1978)	54	17
Bleomycin *Cisplatin*	Vogl (1979)	9	89
Methotrexate *Bleomycin* *Cyclophosphamide*	Lira-Puerto (1979)	70	31
Methotrexate *Adriamycin* *Vincristine*	Bond (1976)	21	48
Adriamycin *Cyclophosphamide* *5-Fluorouracil*	Piver (1978)	15	30
Methotrexate *Vincristine* *Hydroxyurea*	Morrow (1973)	15	6
Bleomycin *Vincristine* *Mitomycin C*	Baker (1976)	30	48 (2CR)
Mitomycin C *Bleomycin* *Vincristine* *Cisplatin*	Alberts (1981)	14	50 (5CR)
Methotrexate *Vincristine* *Bleomycin* *Cisplatin*	Rosenthal (1979)	7	58
Methotrexate *Bleomycin* *Vincristine* *Adriamycin*	Latief (1982)	5	0
Cisplatin *Vincristine* *Mitomycin C*	Vogl (1980)	13	77
BCNU *Vincristine* *Methotrexate* *5-Fluorouracil*	Omura (1973)	7	71
Adriamycin *Vincristine* *Actinomycin D* *Cyclophosphamide*	Piver (1978)	4	0

Table 15.2—continued

Agent	Source	No. of patients	% Objective regression
Cyclophosphamide Actinomycin D 5-Fluorouracil Vincristine Cytosine arabinoside Methotrexate Bleomycin	Forney (1975)	18	50

References

Alberts, D. S., Ignoffo, R., Adriamycin—cyclophosphamide treatment of squamous cell carcinoma of the cervix. *Tumor*, 1976, **62**, 113–22.

Alberts, D. S., Surwit, E. A., Mitomycin C, bleomycin, vincristine and cisplatin in the treatment of advanced recurrent squamous cell carcinoma of the cervix. *Third NCI-EORTC Symposium on New Drugs in Cancer Therapy*, Institut Jules Bordet, Brussels, Belgium, Oct. 15–17, 1981, Abstract No. 10.

Ansfield, F. J., Schroeder, J. M., Curreri, A. R., Five years clinical experience with 5-fluorouracil. *J. Am. Med. Ass.*, 1962, **181**, 295–9.

Baker, L. H., Opipari, M. I., Izbicki, M., Phase II study of mitomycin C, vincristine and bleomycin in advanced squamous carcinoma of the uterine cervix. *Cancer*, 1976, **38**, 2222–4.

Barlow, J. J., Piver, M. S., Chuang, J. T., Cortes, E. P., Ohnuma, T., Holland, J. F., Adriamycin and bleomycin alone, and in combination, in gynecologic cancers. *Cancer*, 1973, **32**, 735–43.

Blaikley, J. B., Lederman, M., O'Connor, K. J., Carcinoma of the cervix at the Chelsea Hospital for Women 1933–60. *Lancet*, 1962, **2**, 978–84.

Blum, R. H., Carter, S. K., Agre, K., A clinical review of bleomycin—a new antineoplastic agent. *Cancer*, 1973, **31**, 903.

Bond, W. H., Holme, G. M., Jones, W. G., Combination chemotherapy in the treatment of advanced squamous cell carcinoma of the cervix. *Clinical Oncology*, 1976, **2**, 173–8.

Bush, R. S., *Malignancies of the ovary, uterus and cervix*. Edward Arnold, 1979, p. 207.

Carlson, J. A., Freedman, R. S., Wallace, S., Chuang, V. P., Wharton, J. T., Rutledge, F. N., Intraarterial cisplatin in the management of squamous carcinoma of the uterine cervix. *Gynecologic Oncology*, 1981, **12**, 92–8.

Carter, S. K., Schabel, F. M., Broder, L. E., Johnston, T. P., 1,3-Bis(2-chloroethyl)-1-nitrosourea (BCNU) and other nitrosoureas in cancer treatment: a review. *Adv. Cancer Res.*, 1972, **16**, 273–332.

Cavins, J. A., Geisler, H. E., Treatment of advanced, unresectable, cervical carcinoma already subjected to complete irradiation therapy. *Gynecol. Oncol.*, 1978, **6**, 256.

Cohen, C. J., Castro-Marin, A., Deppe, G., Chemotherapy of advanced recurrent cervical cancer with cisplatinum (II): a preliminary report. *Proc. Am. Soc. Clin. Oncol.*, 1978, **19**, 401.

Conroy, J. F., Lewis, G. C., Brady, L. W., Brodsky, I., Kahn, S. B., Ross, D., Nuss, R., Low dose bleomycin and methotrexate in cervical cancer. *Cancer*, 1976, **37**, 660–4.

Conroy, J., Lewis, G. C., Brady, L. W., Mangen, C., Hutch, K., Wilbanks, G., Phase II trial of ICRF-159 in treatment of advanced squamous carcinoma of the cervix. *Proc. ASCO*, 1980, **21**, 423.

Day, T. G., Jr., Wharton, J. T., Gottlieb, J. A., Rutledge, F. N., Chemotherapy for squamous carcinoma of the cervix: doxorubicin–methylCCNU. *Am. J. Obstet. Gynecol.*, 1978, **132**, 545–8.

De Palo, G. M., Bajetta, E., Luciani, L., Musumeci, R., di Re, F., Bonadonna, G., Methotrexate (NSC-125066) in the treatment of advanced epidermoid carcinoma of the uterine cervix. *Cancer Chemother. Rep.*, 1973, **57**, 429.

De Vita, V. T. Jr., Wasserman, T. H., Young, R. C., Carter, S. K., Perspectives on research in Gynecologic Oncology. *Cancer*, 1976, **38**, 509–25.

Forney, J. P., Morrow, C. P., Di Saia, P. J., Futoran, R. J., Seven drug polychemotherapy in the treatment of advanced and recurrent squamous carcinoma of the female genital tract. *Am. J. Obstet. Gynecol.*, 1975, **123**, 7, 748–52.

Goldsmith, M. A., Freidman, M. A., Carter, S. K., *DTIC Clinical Brochure* 1972, National Cancer Institute.

Greenberg, B. R., Kardinal, C. G., Pajak, T. F., Bateman, R., Adriamycin versus adriamycin and bleomycin in advanced epidermoid carcinoma of the cervix. *Cancer Treat. Rep.*, 1977, Vol. **61**, 1383–4.

Guthrie, D., Way, S., The use of adriamycin and methotrexate in carcinoma of the cervix. *Obstet. Gynecol.*, 1978, **52**, 349–54.

Haid, M., Homesley, H., White, D. R., Adriamycin–methotrexate combination chemotherapy of advanced carcinoma of the cervix. *Obstet. Gynecol.*, 1977, **50**, 103–5.

Hakes, T., Nikurui, M., Magill, G., Ochoa, M., Cervix cancer—treatment with combination vincristine and high doses of methotrexate. *Cancer*, 1979, **43**, 459–64.

Hall, D. J., Diasio, R., Goplerud, D. R., Cisplatin in Gynecologic Cancer. *Am. J. Obstet. Gynecol.*, 1981, **141**, 305–8.

Hill, G. B., *World Health Statistics Report*, 1975, **28**, 323.

Holland, J. F., Saharlon, C., Gailani, S., Krant, M. J., Olson, K. B., Horton, J., Shnider, B. I., Lynch, J. J., Owens, A., Carbone, P. P., Colsky, J., Grob, D., Miller, S. P., Hall, T. C., Vincristine treatment of advanced cancer: A cooperative study of 392 cases. *Cancer Res.*, 1973, **33**, 1258–64.

Hreshschyshyn, M., Vincristine treatment of patients with carcinoma of the uterine cervix. *Proc. Amer. Assoc. Cancer Res.*, 1963, **4**, 29.

Jolles, B., Long term results of treatment of carcinoma of the cervix. *Br. J. Obstet. Gynae.*, 1980, **87**, 315–21.

Jorgensen, S.-J., Time dose relationships in combined bleomycin treatment and radiotherapy. *European Jr. Cancer*, 1972, **8**, 531–4.

Kottmeier, H. L. *Annual reports on the results of treatment in carcinoma of the uterus, vagina and ovary.* Vol. 16, Stockholm, Pago Print, 1976.

Latief, T. N., Chemotherapy of carcinoma of the cervix—collected cases at the Royal Marsden Hospital, London. 1982, personal communication.

Lederman, M., The treatment of carcinoma of the cervix. *Br. J. Radiol.*, 1964, **37**, 745–7.

Leichman, L. P., Baker, L. H., Stanhope, C. R., Samson, M. K., Fraile, R. J., Vaitkevicius, V. K., Hilgers, R., Mitomycin C and bleomycin in the treatment of far-advanced cervical cancer—a South West Oncology Group pilot study. *Cancer Treat. Rep.*, 1980, **64**, 1139–40.

Lira-Puerto, V. M., Hidalgo, I. N., Morales, F. R., Tenoris, F., Bleomycin, methotrexate, cyclophosphamide in advanced squamous carcinoma of the cervix. *Proc. ASCO*, 1979, **20**, 319.

Malkasian, G. D., Decker, D. G., Mussey, E., Johnson, C. E., Chemotherapy of squamous cell carcinoma of the cervix, vagina and vulva. *Clin. Obstet. Gynec.*, 1968, **11**, 367.

Malkasian, G. D., Decker, D. G., Jorgensen, E. O., Chemotherapy of carcinoma of the cervix. *Gynecologic Oncology*, 1977, **5**(2), 109–20.

Masterson, J. G., Nelson, J. H., The role of chemotherapy in the treatment of gynecologic malignancy. *Am. J. Obstet. Gynecol.*, 1965, **93**, 1102.

Miyamoto, T., Takabe, Y., Watanake, M., Terasima, T., Effectiveness of a sequential combination of bleomycin and mitomycin C on an advanced cervical cancer. *Cancer*, 1978, **41**, 403–14.

Moore, G. E., Bross, I. D. J., Ausman, R., Nadler, S., Jones, R. Jr., Slack, N., Rimm, A. A., Effects of 5-fluorouracil (NSC-19893) in 389 patients with cancer. Eastern Clinical Drug Evaluation Program. *Cancer Chemother. Rep.*, 1968a, **52**, 641–53.

Moore, G. E., Bross, I. D. J., Ausman, R., Nadler, S., Jones, R. Jr., Slack, N., Rimm, A. A., Effects of 6-mercaptopurine (NSC-755) in 290 patients with advanced cancer. *Cancer Chemother. Rep.*, 1968b, **52**(6), 655–60.

Moore, G. E., Bross, I. D. J., Ausman, R., Nadler, S., Jones, R. Jr., Slack, N., Rimm, A. A., Effects of chlorambucil (NSC-3088) in 374 patients with advanced cancer. *Cancer Chemother. Rep.*, 1968c, **52**, 661–84.

Moore, G. E., Bross, I. D. J., Ausman, R., Nadler, S., Jones, R. Jr., Slack, N., Rimm, A. A., Effects of mitomycin C (NSC-19893) in 346 patients with advanced cancer. Eastern Clinical Drug Evaluation Program. *Cancer Chemother. Rep.*, 1968d, **52**, 675–84.

Morrow, C. P., Di Saia, P. J., Mangan, C. F., Lagasse, L. D., Continuous pelvic arterial infusion with bleomycin for squamous carcinoma of the cervix recurrent after irradiation therapy. *Cancer Treat. Rep.*, 1977, **61**(7), 1403–5.

Mould, R. F., Staffurth, J. F., Carcinoma of the cervix at the Royal Marsden Hospital 1962–70: survival results. *Brit. J. Radiol.*, 1979, **52**, 157–8.

Ohnuma, T., Holland, J. F., Masuda, H., Microbiological assay of bleomycin: activation, tissue distribution and clearance. *Cancer*, 1974, **33**, 1230.

Omura, G. A., Chemotherapy and hormone therapy in gynecologic cancer. *South. Med. J.*, 1973, **66**, 689–92.

Papavasiliou, C., Angelakis, P., Gouvalis, P., Papakyriakides, L., Treatment of cervical carcinoma by methotrexate (NSC-740) combined with cyclophosphamide (NSC-26271). *Cancer Chemother. Rep.*, 1969, **53**, 255–61.

Papavasiliou, C., Pappas, J., Ararantinos, D., Kaskarelis, D., Treatment of cervical carcinoma with adriamycin combined with methotrexate. *Cancer Treat. Rep.*, 1978, **62**, 1387–8.

Piel, I. J., Slayton, R. E., Perlia, C. P., Wilbanks, G. D., Combination chemotherapy with bleomycin and methotrexate in recurrent and disseminated cervical carcinoma: a preliminary study. *Gynecol. Oncol.*, 1973, **1**, 184–90.

Piver, M. S., Barlow, J. J., Vontgama, V., Webster, J., Hydroxyurea and radiation therapy in advanced cervical cancer. *Am. J. Obstet. Gynecol.*, 1974, **120**, 969–72.

Piver, M. S., Barlow, J. J., Xynos, F. P., Adriamycin alone or in combination in 100 patients with carcinomas of the cervix or vagina. *Am. J. Obstet. Gynecol.*, 1978, **131**, 311–13.

Powles, R. L., Morgenstern, G., Clink, H. M., Hedley, D., Bandini, G., Lumley, H., Watson, J. G., Lawson, D., Spence, D., Barrett, A., Jameson, B., Lawler, S., Kay, H. E., McElwain, J. L., The place of bone marrow transplantation in acute myelogenous leukaemia. *Lancet*, 1980, **1**, 1047–50.

Rosenthal, C. J., Platica, O., Khulpatua, N., Boyce, J., Alfonso, A., Effective combination chemotherapy of advanced cervical cancer with cisplatin, bleomycin, vincristine, mitomycin C-BOMP. *Proc. AACR*, 1980, **21**, 189.

Roy, D. K., Treatment of advanced or recurrent carcinoma of the cervix by cytotoxic drugs. *Indian J. Cancer*, 1967, **4**, 32–7.

Slavik, M., Adriamycin (NSC-123127) activity in genitourinary and gynecologic malignancies. *Cancer Chemotherapy Rep.*, 1975, Part 3, **6** (Part 2), 277–303.

Slayton, R. E., Mladineo, J., Adriamycin and cisdiamminedichloroplatinum in recurrent and metastatic squamous cell carcinoma of the cervix: a pilot study. *Proc. ASCO*, 1978, **19**, 335.

Slayton, R., Creasman, W., Petty, W., Bundy, B., Blessing, J., Phase II trial of VP-16-213 in the treatment of advanced squamous cell carcinoma of the cervix, and adenocarcinoma of the ovary: a Gynecologic Oncology Group study. *Cancer Treat. Rep.*, 1979, **63**, 2089–92.

Smith, J. P., Rutledge, F., Burns, B. C., Soffar, S., Systemic chemotherapy for carcinoma of the cervix. *Am. J. Obstet. Gynecol.*, 1967, **97**, 800–7.

Solidaro, A. S., Esteves, L., Castellano, C., Valdivia, E., Barriga, O., Chemotherapy of advanced cancer of the cervix: Experience in 55 cases treated with cyclophosphamide. *Am. J. Obstet. Gynecol.*, 1966, **94**, 208–13.

Stolinsky, D. C., Hum, G. J., Jacobs, E. M., Soloman, J., Bateman, J. R., Clinical trial of weekly doses of vinblastine (NSC-49842) combined with vincristine (NSC-67574) in malignant lymphoma and other neoplasms. *Cancer Chemother. Rep.*, 1973, **57**, 477–80.

Suzuki, M., Murai, A., Watanabe, T., Nunokawa, O., Treatment of cancer of the female genital organs with a new anticancer agent bleomycin (BLM). *Acta Med. Biol. (Niigata)*, 1970, **17**, 259–75.

Swenerton, K. D., Evers, J. A., White, G. W., Boyes, D. A., Intermittent pelvic infusion with vincristine, bleomycin and mitomycin C for advanced recurrent carcinoma of the cervix. *Cancer Treat. Rep.*, 1979, **63**(8), 1379–81.

Thigpen, T., Shingleton, H., Phase II trial of cisplatin in treatment of advanced squamous cell carcinoma of the cervix. *ASCO abstracts*, 1978, C-102.

Thigpen, T., Vance, R. B., Balducci, L., Blessing, J., Chemotherapy in the management of advanced or recurrent cervical and endometrial carcinoma. *Cancer*, 1981, **48**, 658–65.

Trussell, R. T., Mitford-Barberton, G. de B., Carcinoma of the cervix treated with continuous intraarterial methotrexate and intramuscular leucovorin. *Lancet*, 1961, **1**, 971–2.

US Dept. of Health, Education and Welfare, 1974. *Recent trends in survival of cancer patients.*

Varga, A., Henriksen, E., Effect of 17-alpha-hydroxyprogesterone 17-n-caproate on various pelvic malignancies. *Obstet. Gynecol.*, 1964, **23**, 51–2.

Vogl, S. E., Moukhtar, M., Kaplan, B. H., Chemotherapy for advanced cervical cancer with methotrexate, bleomycin and cisdiamminedichloroplatinum(II). *Cancer Treat. Rep.*, 1979, **63**, 1005–6.

Vogl, S. E., Moukhtar, M., Kaplan, B. H., Colanog, A., Effective combination chemotherapy of advanced cervical cancer with cisplatin, bleomycin, vincristine, mitomycin C-BOMP. *Proc. AACR*, 1980, **21**, 189.

Wallace, H. J., Jr., Hreshchyshyn, M. M., Wilbanks, G. D., Boronow, R. C., Fowler, W. C. Jr., Blessing, J. A., Comparison of the therapeutic effects of adriamycin alone versus adriamycin plus vincristine versus adriamycin plus cyclophosphamide in the treatment of advanced carcinoma of the cervix. *Cancer Treat. Rep.*, 1978, **62**, 1435–41.

Wasserman, T. H., Slavik, M., Carter, S. K., Review of CCNU in clinical cancer therapy. *Cancer Treat. Rev.*, 1974a, **1**, 131–51.

Wasserman, T. H., Slavik, M., Carter, S. K., Methyl-CCNU in clinical cancer therapy. *Cancer Treat. Rev.*, 1974b, **1**, 251–69.

Wasserman, T. H., Carter, S. K., The integration of chemotherapy into combined modality treatment of solid tumours—VIII cervical cancer. *Cancer Treat. Rev.*, 1977, **4**, 25–46.

Wilson, W. L., Bisel, H. F., Cole, D., Rochlin, D., Ramirez, G., Madden, R., Prolonged low dosage administration of hexamethylmelamine (NCI-3875). *Cancer*, 1970, **25**, 568–70.

Chapter Sixteen

Carcinoma of the Fallopian Tube

Primary adenocarcinoma of the Fallopian tube (uterine) is extremely rare. Only about 1000 cases have been reported. The first case of this tumour was presented by Renaud at a Manchester Pathological Society meeting in 1847 (Doran 1896), but Orthmann gave the first authentic description in 1888. Two hundred and thirty two cases were reviewed by Sedlis in 1961, up to 1955, and Schiller and Silverberg (1971) reviewed 76 cases between 1955 and 1976. Twenty two cases (1955–80) seen at the Royal Marsden Hospital, London, were reported by Raju et al. (1981), and 15 (1968–79) at the University of Washington, Seattle, by Tamimi and Figge (1981), who emphasised the frequency of lymphatic involvement—53% of their cases showed para-aortic node involvement even when disease appeared limited to the tube.

Compared to carcinoma of the ovary, carcinoma of the Fallopian tube seems to present more frequently as early stage disease which may explain the overall 5 year survival figure of approximately 48% of Raju et al. (1981), and 40% of Tamimi and Figge (1981). Extension outside the uterine tube is associated with a survival rate of only 33%. Recurrence rate of 50% for stage I disease is generally reported.

Most patients are treated with total hysterectomy and bilateral salpingo-oophorectomy, if possible. Although there is little evidence to show any advantage in giving postoperative radiotherapy, Benedet et al. (1977) recommend pelvic irradiation including the para-aortic lymph nodes, and the use of intraperitoneal radioactive chromic phosphate in cases where no macroscopic disease is present in the peritoneal cavity. Phelps and Chapman (1974) held similar views.

There are few data available on the use of chemotherapy in this condition. Treatment of recurrent disease has proved difficult and, in view of the early dissemination, 'adjuvant' postoperative chemotherapy may well be desirable. Raju et al. (1981) treated patients with recurrent disease using cisplatin—one patient entered a complete remission and another showed a partial response. A patient with stage I disease was given chlorambucil for two years following postoperative radiotherapy and had a continuing tumour-free survival in excess of 5 years. No response in recurrent disease was produced using a combination of cyclophosphamide, vincristine and 5-fluorouracil, or single agent hexamethylmelamine. Tamimi and Figge (1981) treated 4 patients with melphalan on an adjuvant basis and were alive without evidence of disease. Of the others treated similarly with single alkylating agents, there was one complete response and the patient was alive without any evidence of disease after 52 months, and two partial responses. Four patients who received combination chemotherapy second line showed no responses. Tamimi and Figge (1981) also questioned the value if any of using progesterone therapy in view of the response of the tubal epithelium to cyclic ovarian hormones. However, Raju et al. (1981) treated three patients with end-stage disease using progestogen therapy and saw no responses.

References

Benedet, J. L., White, G. W., Fairey, R. N., Boyes, D. A., Adenocarcinoma of the Fallopian Tube. *Obstet. Gynecol.*, 1977, **50**, 654.

Doran, A., Preliminary cancer of the Fallopian tube. *Trans. Obstet. Soc. London*, 1896, **38**, 322–6.

Orthmann, E. C., Ueber Primäres Tubencarcinom. *Z. Geburt. Gynek.*, 1888, **15**, 212–24.

Phelps, H. M., Chapman, K. E., Role of radiotherapy in the treatment of primary carcinoma of the uterine tube. *Obstet. Gynecol.*, 1974, **43**, 669–73.

Raju, K. S., Barker, G. H., Wiltshaw, E., Primary carcinoma of the Fallopian tube. *Br. J. Obstet. Gynae.*, 1981, 1124–9.

Schiller, H. M., Silverberg, S. G., Staging and prognosis in primary carcinoma of the Fallopian tube. *Cancer*, 1971, **28**, 389–95.

Sedlis, A., Primary carcinoma of the Fallopian tube. *Obstetric and Gynecological Survey*, 1961, **16**, 209–26.

Tamimi, H. K., Figge, D. C., Adenocarcinoma of the uterine tube: potential for lymph node metastases. *Am. J. Obstet. Gynecol.*, 1981, **141**, 132–7.

Chapter Seventeen

Carcinoma of the Endometrium

The use of nonhormonal chemotherapy in carcinoma of the endometrium, the third most common cause of death from gynaecological malignancy, is not widespread. Few large scale series have been reported. The majority of women have well differentiated early stage lesions and the overall cure rate is relatively high—approximately 70% (Thigpen et al. 1981), especially as significant prognostic factors are histological differentiation and the extent of spread at diagnosis.

Table 17.1 Single agents in the management of advanced or recurrent endometrial carcinoma

Agent	Source	No. of patients	Objective response
5-Fluorouracil	Moore (1968)	8	2PR
	De Vita (1976)	43	23%
	Donovan (1974)		25%
6-Mercaptopurine	Moore (1968)	2	0
Cyclophosphamide	Donovan (1974)		28%
	De Vita (1976)	33	21%
	Horton (1978)	19	0
Chlorambucil	Moore (1968)	6	0
Cisplatin	Thigpen (1981)	25	4%
	Loeb (1975)	2	2PR
	Deppe (1980)	13	2PR
Methyl-CCNU	Omura (1978)	6	33%
Adriamycin	Monson (1972)	18	39%
	Thigpen (1979)	43	37%
	De Vita (1976)	18	38%
	Horton (1978)	21	19%
Mitomycin C	Moore (1968)	2	1PR
Piperazinedione	La Gasse (1979)	20	5%

However, the prognosis for late stage and recurrent early stage disease is poor (Kottmeier 1976):

5 year survival of endometrial carcinoma

Stage I—76%

II—50%

III—30%

IV— 9%

The incidence of vaginal recurrence after treatment of stage I disease is variously given as between 3% and 11% depending on tumour differentiation, and the incidence of lymph node metastases is to a large extent related to the degree of myometrial invasion. Metastatic spread, eg to the lungs, may be extensive and in excess of that easily treated by radiotherapy.

There are thus several areas in the management of this condition where systemic chemotherapy may have a role. Tables 17.1 and 17.2 give a summary of the few studies to date.

Table 17.2 Combination chemotherapy in the management of advanced or recurrent endometrial carcinoma

Agent	Source	No. of patients	Objective response
Adriamycin *Cyclophosphamide*	Muggia (1977)	8	75% (3CR, 2PR)
Adriamycin *Cyclophosphamide* *Cisplatin*	Koretz (1980)	7	56%
Melphalan *5-Fluorouracil* *Medroxy-progesterone-* *acetate*	Piver (1980) Cohen (1977)	11 15	54% 93%
Adriamycin *Cyclophosphamide* *5-Fluorouracil* *Medroxy-progesterone-* *acetate*	Bruckner (1977)	20	75%

Hormone therapy

Since the early 1950s a variety of hormone preparations have been shown to be helpful in this condition. Glassburn (1981) reports the response rate of endometrial carcinoma to progestational agents as lying between 20% and 50%. Bonte et al. (1978) reported the elimination of in situ endometrial carcinoma in 62% of all cases and 30% of invasive tumours using medroxyprogesterone acetate, and a remission rate of 53% in disseminated or recurrent disease.

Reifenstein (1971) induced widespread tumour reduction with hydroxy-progesterone caproate in 30% of patients.

Creasman et al. (1980) demonstrated that patients without oestrogen or progesterone receptors in their tumour failed to respond to progestogen therapy.

Karlstedt (1972) suggests that those responding favourably to hormone therapy are those who are young with well differentiated tumours and a long disease free interval after initial treatment, although Bush (1979) denies that age is influential.

Bonte et al. (1978) claimed marked enhancement of survival of Stage I (via a radiosensitisation of the tumour) by adjuvant hormone therapy both prior to, and following, radiosurgical treatment. However, Lewis et al. (1974) could not demonstrate any improvement using hormone therapy preoperatively in stage I disease. Approaching the problem in the opposite way the antioestrogen tamoxifen is currently being studied in the management of this tumour (Swenerton et al. 1979).

References

Bonte, J., Decoster, J. M., Ide, P., Billiet, G., Hormone prophylaxis and hormonotherapy in the treatment of endometrial adenocarcinoma by means of medroxyprogesterone acetate. *Gynecologic Oncology*, 1978, **6**, 60–75.

Bruckner, H. W., Deppe, G., Combination chemotherapy of advanced endometrial adenocarcinoma with adriamycin, cyclophosphamide, 5-fluorouracil and medroxy-progesterone acetate. *Obstet. Gynecol.*, 1977, **50**, 105–25.

Bush, R. S. *Malignancies of the ovary, uterus and cervix*, Edward Arnold, 1979, p. 132.

Cohen, C. J., Deppe, G., Bruckner, H. W., Treatment of advanced adenocarcinoma of the endometrium with melphalan, 5-fluorouracil and medroxyprogesterone acetate. *Obstet. Gynaecol.*, 1977, **50**, 415–17.

Creasman, W. T., McCarty, K. S., Barton, T. K., McCarty, K. S. Jr., Clinical correlates of estrogen and progesterone binding proteins in human endometrial adenocarcinoma. *Obstet. Gynecol.*, 1980, **55**, 363–70.

De Vita, V. T. Jr., Wasserman, T. H., Young, R. C., Carter, S. K., Prospectives on research in gynaecologic oncology. *Cancer*, 1976, **38**, 509–25.

Deppe et al. In Cisplatin in the treatment of cervical and endometrial cancer patients; Baker, L. H. In *Cisplatin: current status and new developments*, ed. Prestayko, A. W., Crooke, S. T., Carter, S. K. Academic Press, New York, 1980, p. 408.

Donovan, J. F., Nonhormonal chemotherapy of endometrial carcinoma. A review. *Cancer*, 1974, **34**, 1587–92.

Glassburn, J. R., Cancer of the endometrium. *Cancer*, 1981, **48**, 579.

Horton, J., Bezz, C. B., Arsenan, J., Bruckner, H., Creech, R., Hahn, R. G., Comparison of adriamycin and cyclophosphamide in patients with advanced endometrial cancer. *Cancer Treatment Rep.*, 1978, **62**, 154–61.

Karlstedt, K., Effect of progesterone on metastases and local recurrences of carcinoma of the uterine corpus. *Acta Obstet. Gynecol., Scand.*, 1972, **19**, 11–12.

Koretz, M. M., Ballon, S., Friedman, M. A., Donaldson, S., Platinum, adriamycin and cyclophosphamide (PAC) chemotherapy in advanced endometrial carcinoma. *Proc. AACR*, 1980, **21**, 195.

Kottmeier, H. L., Annual reports on the results of treatment in carcinoma of the uterus, vagina and cervix. **16**, Stockholm, Pago Print, 1976.

La Gasse, L., Thigpen, T., Morrison, F. S., Phase II trial of piperazinedione in the treatment of advanced endometrial carcinoma, uterine sarcoma, vulval carcinoma. *Proc. ASCO*, 1979, **20**, 388.

Lewis, G. C., Slack, N. H., Mortel, R., Bross, I. D. J., Adjuvant progestogen therapy in the primary definitive treatment of endometrial cancer. *Gynecologic Oncology*, 1974, **2**, 368–76.

Loeb, E., Hill, J. M., MacLellan, A., Hill, N. O., Khan, A., King, J. J., Speer, R., Ridgeway, H. *Wadley Medical Bulletin*, 1975, **5**, 281–93.

Monson, R. R., MacMahon, B., Austin, J. H., When may endometrial cancer be considered cured? *Cancer*, 1972, **30**, 419–25.

Moore, G. E., Bross, I. D. J., Ausman, R., Nadler, S., Jones, R., Slack, N., Rimm, A. A., Effects of 5-fluorouracil, 6-mercaptopurine, chlorambucil and mitomycin C in patients with cancer. *Cancer Chemother. Rep.* (Part 1), 1968, **52**, 641.

Muggia, F. M., Chia, G., Reed, L. J., Romney, S. L., Doxorubicin—cyclophosphamide: effective chemotherapy for advanced endometrial adenocarcinoma. *Am. J. Obstet. Gynecol.*, 1977, **128**, 314–18.

Omura, G. A., Shingleton, H. M., Creasman, W. T., Blessing, J. A., Boronow, R. C., Chemotherapy of gynecologic cancer with nitrosoureas: a randomised trial of CCNU and methyl-CCNU in cancers of the cervix, corpus, vagina and vulva. *Cancer Treat. Rep.*, 1978, **62**, 833.

Piver, M. S., Lele, S., Barlow, J. J., Melphalan, 5-fluorouracil and medroxyprogesterone acetate in metastatic endometrial carcinoma. *Proc. ASCO 1980*, **21**, 425.

Reifenstein, E. C. Jr., Hydroxyprogesterone caproate therapy in advanced endometrial cancer. *Cancer*, 1971, **27**, 485–502.

Swenerton, K. D., White, G. W., Boyes, D. A., Treatment of advanced endometrial carcinoma with tamoxifen. *New Engl. J. Med.*, 1979, **301**, 105.

Thigpen, T., Bushsbaum, H. J., Mangan, C., Blessing, J. A., Phase II trial of adriamycin in the treatment of advanced or recurrent endometrial carcinoma; a Gynecologic Oncology Group study. *Cancer Treat. Rep.*, 1979, **63**, 21–27.

Thigpen, T., Vance, R. B., Balducci, L., Blessing, J., Chemotherapy in the management of advanced or recurrent cervical and endometrial carcinoma. *Cancer*, 1981, **48**, 658–65.

Chapter Eighteen

Vaginal Tumours

Primary vaginal tumours are relatively rare. Since the majority consist of squamous cell carcinomas, what few reports there are of these tumours being treated by chemotherapy are usually included in data for carcinoma of the cervix. Genital tract rhabdomyosarcoma is dealt with separately in Chapter 21. Primary malignant melanomas are occasionally reported. Endodermal sinus tumours of the vagina, for example, are exceedingly rare, with less than 20 cases reported in the literature (Rezaizadeh and Woodruff 1978).

Clinical appearances may be deceptive—the endodermal sinus tumour may resemble sarcoma botryoides or may be confused with the clear cell carcinoma described later. Endodermal sinus tumours of the vagina probably arise from aberrant germ cells distributed along the midline of the body in embryonic life. Radiation, in the case described by Rezaizadeh and Woodruff (1978), and by others, was unhelpful (Alleyn et al. 1971). In view of the interest in the chemotherapy of endodermal sinus tumours of the ovary, a correct histological diagnosis should be made, and chemotherapy considered if necessary.

There are no large trials of chemotherapy in squamous cell carcinomas of the vagina and no clear evidence of activity by any agents, as yet, either single or multiple. Omura et al. (1978) treated three patients with CCNU and two with methyl CCNU and produced no response. Hall et al. (1981) treated one patient aged 38 years with a recurrent squamous cell carcinoma of the vagina several years after hysterectomy for carcinoma in situ of the cervix using cisplatin and produced a brief partial response.

Carcinoma in situ

Since the early 1960s there has been a steady and increasing flow of reports in the literature recording the finding of vaginal carcinoma in situ (Scokel et al. 1961). Woodruff et al. (1975) noted that cases with carcinoma in situ of the vagina appeared to be increasing and that therapy in the past had consisted of either radiotherapy or surgery, ie partial or total vaginectomy, followed in some cases by plastic surgery to reconstruct a vaginal canal. They pointed out that radiotherapy may reduce the plasticity of the vaginal tissues, interfering with sexual intercourse, and that examples were known of recurrent neoplasia in either the surgically restored or the irradiated vagina. They therefore treated nine patients (1968–75) at Johns Hopkins Hospital, Baltimore, with vaginal carcinoma in situ using topical 5-fluorouracil. Only one failed to respond and this patient was subsequently successfully treated by vaginectomy, the remainder being rendered free of disease and followed for up to 6 years without recurrence.

Clear cell carcinoma of the vagina

The association between maternal diethylstilboestrol therapy and the development of clear cell adenocarcinoma of the vagina in young women is well known (Herbst et al. 1971); of 154 young women with clear cell adenocarcinoma of the genital tract the recurrence rate after initial therapy was 21% of 89 with vaginal primaries, and 28% of 65 with cervical primaries, and in the 37 cases with recurrent disease initial treatment with chemotherapy alone was used in 3 cases and combined chemoradiotherapy in another three cases. Nine cases had radiation alone and the remainder were given surgery varying in extent from local excision to pelvic exenteration (Robboy et al. 1974). Twenty four of the 37 patients died 6 to 68 months after initial treatment of the primary tumour, and only 6 of those alive were thought to be tumour free. After 15 drugs were used singly or in combination in 32 trials for the treatment of primary, persistent or recurrent tumour, it was thought that the vinca alkaloids and 5-fluorouracil were beneficial in a few instances. Five cases were treated with progestational agents and received no benefit. The correct successful management of these special tumours in every case has not yet been achieved—the role of chemotherapy should be explored further in view of the failure, in a significant proportion of cases, of surgery and/or radiotherapy to produce total cure.

References

Alleyn, D. L., Silverberg, S. G., Salzberg, A. M., Endodermal sinus tumour of vagina. Report of a case with 7 years survival and review of the so-called 'mesonephromas'. *Cancer*, 1971, **27**, 1231–8.

Hall, D. J., Diasio, R., Goplerud, D. R., Cisplatin in gynecologic cancer II. Squamous cell carcinoma of the cervix. *Am. J. Obstet. Gynecol.*, 1981, **141**, 305.

Herbst, A. L., Ulfeder, H., Poskanzer, D. C., Adenocarcinoma of the vagina. Association of maternal stilboestrol therapy with tumor appearance in young women. *N. Engl. J. Med.*, 1971, **284**, 878–81.

Omura, G. A., Shingleton, H. M., Creasman, W. T., Blessing, J. A., Boronow, R. C., Chemotherapy and gynecologic cancer with nitrosoureas: A randomised trial of CCNU and methyl CCNU in cancers of the cervix, corpus, vagina and vulva. *Cancer Treat. Rep.*, 1978, **62**, 833.

Rezaizadeh, M. M., Woodruff, J. D., Endodermal sinus tumour of vagina. *Gynecologic Oncology*, 1978, **6**, 459–63.

Robboy, S. J., Herbst, A. L., Scully, R. E., Clear cell adenocarcinoma of the vagina and cervix in young females. *Cancer*, 1974, **34**, 606–14.

Scokel, P. W., Collier, F. C., Jones, W. N., McMannus, J. F. A., Hutchins, K., Relation of carcinoma in-situ of the vagina to the early diagnosis of vaginal cancer. *Am. J. Obstet. Gynecol.*, 1961, **82**, 397.

Woodruff, J. D., Parmley, T. H., Julian, C. G., Topical 5-fluorouracil in the treatment of vaginal carcinoma in situ. *Gynecologic Oncology*, 1975, **3**, 124–32.

Chapter Nineteen

Carcinoma of the Vulva

Cancer of the vulva (squamous carcinoma, malignant melanoma, endodermal sinus tumours, sarcomas etc.) accounts for approximately 5% of all primary gynaecological malignancies. Spread to the lymph nodes is common and its occurrence is relative to tumour size. Forty per cent or more of patients have disease in the lymph nodes when the tumour exceeds 3 cm in diameter. Conversely, only 8% of microinvasive lesions were associated with lymph node metastases (Tamimi 1980). The incidence of recurrence in surgically resectable cases is 20% (Masterson and Nelson 1965).

Although Krupp et al. (1976) produced some success in very advanced (Stage IV) vulval carcinoma using ultraradical surgery, in those patients who were over 71 years the results were dismal, with no survivors among those treated with radical vulvectomy, exenteration and lymphadenectomy. This is an obvious area of the disease where chemotherapy may well make a valuable contribution. Indeed, Yahia et al. (1978) in Boston, produced a 42 month palliative response in an 84 year old presenting with a huge vulval cancer fixed to the bone, using a combination of partial excision and twice weekly bleomycin.

In-situ vulval carcinoma

The procedures for vulvectomy, even with conservation techniques such as the 'skinning vulvectomy' and skin grafting, are still frightening and unpleasant surgical procedures especially for those patients who are relatively young.

Buscema et al. (1980) reported that out of 102 such patients followed up to 15 years only 4 developed invasive cancer after vulvectomy or wide local excision. Chemotherapy, either topical or systemic, may well be suitable for this condition and prevent unnecessary surgery. Most experience has been with 5-fluorouracil but there has also been research into other substances such as dinitrochlorobenzene which is thought to act immunologically (Foster and Woodruff 1980).

Sillman et al. (1980) have shown promising results using colposcopically directed excisional biopsies performed while the vulval epithelium is under the influence of topical 5-fluorouracil, followed by monthly 5-fluorouracil maintenance therapy—again obviating the need for mutilating surgery for very early disease, especially in premenopausal women.

Table 19.1   Single agent chemotherapy for carcinoma of the vulva

Agent	Source	No. of patients	Objective response
Cyclophosphamide	Malkasian (1968)		
	Frick (1965)	2	0
Cytembena	Dvorak (1971)	26	4
CCNU	Omura (1978)	4	0
Methyl-CCNU	Omura (1978)	3	0
5-Fluorouracil	Masterson (1965)	2	0
Methotrexate	Deppe (1979)	5	2
6-Mercaptopurine	Masterson (1965)	1	0
Mitomycin C	Masterson (1965)	1	0
Adriamycin	Barlow (1973)	2	1
	Deppe (1977)	4	3
Bleomycin	Deppe (1979)	31	19
	Tropé (1980)	11	5
	Edsmyr (1972)	3	2

Table 19.2   Combination chemotherapy for squamous cell carcinoma of the vulva

Agent	Source	No. of patients	Objective response
Bleomycin Methotrexate	Mosher (1972)	1	1
Bleomycin Mitomycin C	Tropé (1980)	9	5
Adriamycin Cisplatin	Vogl (1976)	1	0
Bleomycin Vincristine Methotrexate	Turner (1975)	7	4
Methotrexate Hydroxyurea Vincristine	Morrow (1973)	2	0
6-Mercaptopurine Thiotepa Melphalan	Frick (1965)	2	0
Cyclophosphamide 5-Fluorouracil Actinomycin D Vincristine Cytosine arabinoside Methotrexate Bleomycin	Forney (1975)	1	1

Advanced and recurrent disease

Way (1960) and Gusberg and Frick (1978) gave 5 year survival rates of patients with unilateral inguinal node involvement of only 40–50%. Postoperative radiotherapy does not appear to be beneficial in such patients (Bachstrom et al. 1972). Inoperable anal and perianal carcinomas have been successfully treated with 5-fluorouracil plus mitomicin C, followed by radiotherapy and surgery (Bruckner et al. 1979). A similar approach was made by Kalva et al. (1981) on two patients with advanced, initially inoperable, vulval cancers, and achieved complete remissions in both and subsequent operability. Table 19.1 gives an appraisal of the published work to date mainly recorded by Deppe et al. (1979), showing the range of activity available for single agents, and Table 19.2 for combination therapy. There are obviously areas in the management of this disease which need to be explored, with the addition or substitution of systemic chemotherapy to established surgical and radiotherapeutic treatments, which are not only distressing to the patient but are clearly inadequate, as shown by the poor survival rates for all but very early disease.

References

Bachstrom, A., Edysmyr, F. et al., Radiotherapy of carcinoma of the vulva. *Acta. Obstet. Gynecol. Scand.*, 1972, **51**, 109.

Barlow, J. J., Piver, M. S., Chueng, J. T., Cortes, E. P., Ohnuma, T., Holland, J. F., Adriamycin and bleomycin, alone and in combination in gynecologic cancers. *Cancer*, 1973, **32**, 735–43.

Bruckner, H. W., Spigelman, M. K., et al., Carcinoma of the anus treated with a combination of radiotherapy and chemotherapy. *Cancer Treat. Rep.*, 1979, **63**, 395–8.

Buscema, J., Woodruff, J. D., Parmley, T. H., Genadry, R., Carcinoma in situ of the vulva. *Obstet. Gynecol.*, 1980, **55**, 255.

Deppe, G., Bruckner, H. W., Cohen, C. J., Adriamycin treatment of advanced vulvar carcinoma. *Obstet. Gynecol.*, 1977, **50**, 135–45.

Deppe, G., Cohen, C. J., Bruckner, H. W., Chemotherapy of squamous cell carcinoma of the vulva: a review. *Gynecologic Oncology*, 1979, **7**, 345–8.

Dvorak, O., Cytembena treatment of advanced gynaecological carcinoma. *Neoplasma*, 1971, **18**, 461–4.

Edsmyr, F., Bleomycin in the treatment of malignant diseases. In *Proceedings of the International Symposium, London, England, Nov. 1972*, pp. 95–103.

Forney, J. P., Morrow, C. P., DiSaia, P. J., Futuran, R. J., Seven drug polychemotherapy in the treatment of advanced and recurrent squamous cell carcinoma of the female genital tract. *Am. J. Obstet. Gynecol.*, 1975, **93**, 1112–21.

Foster, D. C., Woodruff, J. D., The use of dinitrochlorobenzene in the treatment of vulvar carcinoma in situ. *Gynecologic Oncology*, 1980, **11**, 330–9.

Frick, H. C., Atchoo, N., Adamsons, K., Taylor, H. C., The efficacy of chemotherapeutic agents in the management of disseminated gynecologic cancer—Review of 206 cases. *Am. J. Obstet. Gynecol.*, 1965, **93**, 1112–21.

Gusberg, S. B., Frick, H. C. *Corscaden's gynecological cancer*, 5th Ed., Williams & Wilkins, Baltimore, 1978.

Kalva, J. K., Grossman, A. M., Krumholz, B. A., Chen, S., Tinker, M. A., Flores, G. T., Molho, L., Cortes, E. P., Preoperative chemoradiotherapy for carcinoma of the vulva. *Gynecologic Oncology*, 1981, **12**, 256–60.

Krupp, P. J., Bohm, J. W., Lee, F. Y., Collins, J. H., Current status of the treatment of epidermoid cancer of the vulva. *Cancer*, 1976, **38**, 587.

Malkasian, G. D., Decker, D. G., Mussey, E., Johnson, C. E., Chemotherapy of squamous cell carcinoma of the cervix, vagina and vulva. *Clin. Obstet. Gynecol.*, 1968, **11**, 367–81.

Masterson, J. G., Nelson, J. H., The role of chemotherapy in the treatment of gynecologic malignancy. *Am. J. Obstet. Gynecol.*, 1965, **93**(8), 1102–11.

Morrow, C. P., Creasman, W. T., DiSaia, P. J., Curry, S. L., De Petrillo, A. D., Methotrexate, hydroxyurea and vincristine: combination chemotherapy in squamous carcinoma of the female genitalia. *Gynecol. Oncol.*, 1973, **1**, 314–19.

Mosher, M. B., Deconti, R. C., Bertino, J. R., Bleomycin therapy in advanced Hodgkin's disease and epidermoid cancer. *Cancer*, 1972, **30**, 56–60.

Omura, G. A., Shingleton, H. M., Creasman, W. T., Boronow, R. C., Chemotherapy of gynaecologic cancer with nitrosoureas: a randomised trial of CCNU and methyl CCNU in cancers of the cervix, corpus, vagina and vulva. *Cancer Treat. Rep.*, 1978, **62**, 833–5.

Sillman, F. H., Boyce, J. G., Macasaet, M. A., Nicastri, A. D., 5-fluorouracil/chemosurgery for intraepithelial neoplasia of the lower genital tract. *Abstracts of the Society of Gynecologic Oncologists*. Florida, Jan 11–13, 1980.

Tamimi, H. K., in *Gynaecologic oncology—controversies in cancer treatment*, ed. Ballon, S. C., 1980, G. K. Hall, Boston, Mass., p. 41.

Tropé, C., Johnsson, J.-E., Larsson, G., Simonsen, E., Bleomycin alone or combined with mitomycin C in the treatment of advanced or recurrent squamous cell carcinoma of the vulva. *Cancer Treat. Rep.*, 1980, **64**, 639–42.

Turner, R., Paper read at the Bleomycin Meeting, Hammersmith Hospital, London, England, Oct. 1975.

Vogl, S., Ohnuma, T., Perloff, M., Holland, J. F., Combination chemotherapy with adriamycin and cisdichlorodiammine platinum (II) in patients with neoplastic disease. *Cancer*, 1976, **38**, 21–6.

Way, S., Carcinoma of the vulva. *Am. J. Obstet. Gynecol.*, 1960, **79**, 692.

Yahia, C., Fuller, A. F., Cloud, L. P., Successful long term palliation of Stage IV vulvar carcinoma with operation and bleomycin sulphate. *Am. J. Obstet. Gynecol.*, 1978, **130**(3), 360–1.

Chapter Twenty

Uterine Sarcoma

This chapter deals with the sarcomas arising from the uterus other than embryonal rhabdomyosarcoma (sarcoma botryoides) which is covered separately in Chapter 21.

The WHO International Classification of Uterine Tumours separates them into leiomyosarcoma, endometrial stromal sarcoma, mixed Mullerian tumours, carcinosarcoma and mixed mesodermal tumours. However, since uterine sarcomas are relatively rare (approximately 4% of primary uterine cancers) reports of their treatment by chemotherapy often include them in a group of 'soft tissue sarcomas' in order to separate them, basically, from osteogenic sarcoma which is, incidentally, relatively chemosensitive.

Nearly all uterine sarcomas, of any stage, offer a gloomy prognosis but of all the soft tissue sarcomas arising in various parts of the body those of uterine origin have, in various trials, responded more frequently than those of other sites.

Because of their rarity large numbers of patients with these tumours have not been treated actively with chemotherapy, but some factors influencing prognosis are apparent.

Firstly, even very early stage tumours which are well excised may have the capacity to metastasise. Buchsbaum et al. (1979), in Iowa City, reported a 7% survival rate for stage I and II leiomyosarcoma with over 5 mitoses per 10 HPF and no patient survived whose tumour contained more than 10 mitoses per 10 HPF. The results were similar with mixed mesodermal tumours and only slightly better with endometrial stromal sarcoma.

Christopherson et al. (1972) were surprised to find great variance in the reported five year survival rates of patients with uterine leiomyosarcoma, ie between none (Bartsich et al. 1968) to 68% (Novak and Anderson 1937) and reviewed 153 cases examined in Jefferson County, Kentucky, between 1953 and 1969. They concluded that mitotic indices were of profound importance. Hart and Billman (1978) indicated that cellular myomas and tumours with fewer than 3 to 5 mitoses per 10 HPF carry a good prognosis while those with over 10 mitoses per 10 HPF were almost always fatal.

Montague et al. (1965) estimated that the incidence of sarcomatous change in leiomyomas was only 0.29%.

The second factor is that recurrence and/or metastases are exceedingly difficult to treat successfully. Yazigi et al. (1979) report a five year survival rate for 224 patients with stage III uterine sarcomas of only 7.1%.

Thirdly, whereas excision of the tumour is accepted as being helpful, the addition of subsequent irradiation does not appear to influence the progress of the disease (Smith 1941). However, after reviewing the literature, Piver and Lurain (1981) concluded that radiotherapy had a role in the combined treatment of malignant Müllerian mixed tumours and endometrial stromal sarcomas confined to the pelvis, by increasing the disease-free progression interval and increasing pelvic control and probably increased overall survival.

Leiomyosarcomas show little, if any, response to radiotherapy. Attention has therefore been given to the possible role for adjuvant chemotherapy based upon agents which are known to cause regression of widespread disease. However, adjuvant chemotherapy has not been shown, as yet, to influence the course of these tumours to any great extent.

Prophylactic chemotherapy

Buchsbaum et al. (1979) treated ten patients with stage I or II disease on a postoperative, adjuvant basis using vincristine, actinomycin D and cyclo-phosphamide (VAC) in 6 courses over 6 months. The results, after between 3 and 7 years of following up all patients, were: five alive without evidence of disease, two dead of intercurrent disease free of tumour, and one alive with disease. Recurrences were treated with high dose methotrexate and later adriamycin but none survived. They cautiously conclude that prophylactic chemotherapy may be effective in reducing recurrence and that since the sites of metastases are commonly outside the pelvis they suggest that radiotherapy confined to the pelvis would not modify the outcome.

In a small prospective study at Roswell Park Memorial Institute, patients with early stage uterine sarcomas were given adjuvant adriamycin versus no adjuvant chemotherapy, following intracavitary radium, total abdominal hysterectomy and bilateral salpingo-oophorectomy. Two patients out of six in each group developed recurrent disease within 12 months and it was concluded that adjuvant adriamycin was of no benefit in early stage disease (Piver and Lurain 1981).

Other studies

Subraminian and Wiltshaw (1978) indicated that soft tissue sarcomas were known to have responded to actinomycin D, cyclophosphamide, vincristine, metho-trexate, adriamycin and dimethyl triazeno imidazol carboxamide (DTIC). However, the complete response rate remained at around 10%. In their report of 75 assessable cases treated with methotrexate alone and in combination with other agents, three patients with uterine leiomyosarcomas showed complete responses (24, 89 and 29 months) to methotrexate alone and one patient with malignant mixed Müllerian tumour to STS (soft tissue sarcoma regimen), ie methotrexate, adriamycin and DTIC, for 18+ months. They concluded on the whole series that although partial regressions may be dramatic they seldom lasted long. Complete responses were uncommon but were often associated with prolonged survival. However, with complete response rates of only 10 to 15%, they did not feel that adjuvant chemotherapy would be useful in the majority of cases. Subsequently, 37 patients with advanced soft tissue sarcomas were treated with STS-II (vincristine, actinomycin D, cyclophosphamide, adriamycin, methotrexate) (Bryant and Wiltshaw 1980), and there were two complete responses and three partial responses. Of the complete responders both sarcomas originated in the uterus (leiomyosarcoma and endometrial stromal sarcoma) and one of the partial responders was also an endometrial stromal sarcoma of uterus.

An interesting feature involved the reports that a multidrug combination CY-VA-DIC (cyclophosphamide vincristine, adriamycin and imidazole carbox-amide) was effective (response rate 60%) in the management of metastatic

Table 20.1 Chemotherapy of uterine sarcomas

Agent(s)	Source	Tumour	No. of patients	Objective response
CCNU	Omura (1978a)		6	1CR
Methyl-CCNU	Omura (1978a)		6	0
Cisplatin	Karakousis (1979)	Leiomyosarcoma		1CR (6 months)
Cisplatin	Thigpen (1980)		20	20% (1CR, 3PR)
Adriamycin	Piver (1979)		17	6%
Adriamycin	Omura (1978b)		51	27%
Adriamycin	Yazigi (1979)	Endometrial stromal sarcoma		1CR (6 years)
Adriamycin DTIC	Omura (1978b)		40	27%
Then VAC	Azizi (1979)	Leiomyosarcoma	6	3CR, 1PR (mean duration of response = 16 months) (1 patient tumour free for 24 months)
Vincristine Actinomycin D Cyclophosphamide	Smith (1975b)	Malignant mixed Müllerian	13	3CR ⎫ tumour
		Leiomyosarcoma	8	7CR ⎬ free 10–56 months
		Endometrial stromal	3	0 ⎭
Adriamycin DTIC +Vincristine	Gottlieb (1972)	Leiomyosarcoma	16	6
VAC or VAD	Creagan (1976)		69	19%, 8%
Adriamycin Cyclophosphamide Vincristine DTIC	Parente (1978)	Leiomyosarcoma	1	1CR (10 months)

sarcomas (Gottlieb et al. 1974); whilst later studies found the same regimen ineffective (response rate 15%) (Giuliano et al. 1978). However, Benjamin et al. (1976) did report on 178 patients treated with CY-VA-DIC (13% CR, 33%PR) and in combination with actinomycin D = CY-VA-DACT (12% CR, 27%PR).

Yoonessi and Hart (1977) greatly emphasise the prognostic difference between uterine endometrial stromatosis and stromal sarcomata. They report that stromal sarcomas have very high mitotic rates (10 to 20 mitoses per 10 HPF) whilst stromatosis generally has less than 5 mitoses per 10 HPF. They report 100% mortality in 9 patients with stromal sarcoma whilst Kempson and Bari (1970), report 100% tumour free survival (3 to 15 years) in patients with stromatosis. Barlow et al. (1973) obtained partial responses in all three of patients with metastatic stromal sarcoma treated with adriamycin. Rosenbaum and Schoenfield (1977) found VAC (vincristine, actinomycin D, and cyclophosphamide) effective in this tumour as did Lehrner et al. (1979), combining VAC with megestrol acetate, and obtaining a complete remission in one patient. Megestrol acetate was added since progestogens have been shown to have activity against metastatic stromal myosis (Krumholz et al. 1973). Smith and Rutledge (1975a) however, did not find VAC as effective.

Table 20.1 demonstrates the attempts to treat metastatic disease with a variety of agents.

References

Azizi, F., Bitran, J., Javehari, G., Herbst, A. L., Remission of uterine leiomyosarcoma treated with vincristine, adriamycin and DTIC. *Am. J. Obstet. Gynecol.*, 1979, **133**, 379.

Barlow, J. J., Piver, M. S., Chuang, J. T., Cortes, E. P., Ohmura, T., Holland, J. F., Adriamycin and bleomycin, alone and in combination, in gynecologic cancers. *Cancer*, 1973, **32**, 735–43.

Bartsich, E. G., Bowe, E. T., Moore, J., Leiomyosarcoma of the uterus: a 50 year review. *Obstet. Gynecol.*, 1968, **32**, 101–6.

Benjamin, R. S., Gottlieb, J. A., Baker, L. O., Sinkovics, J. G., A randomised trial of cyclophosphamide (CY), vincristine (V), adriamycin (A) plus dacarbazine (DIC) or actinomycin D (DACT). *Proc. Am. Assoc. Cancer Res. and ASCO*, 1976, **17**, 256.

Bryant, B. M., Wiltshaw, E., Results of the Royal Marsden Hospital Second Soft Tissue Sarcoma Schedule (STS-II) chemotherapy regimen in the management of advanced sarcoma. *Cancer Treat. Rep.*, 1980, **64**, 4–5, 609–92.

Buchsbaum, H. J., Lifshitz, S., Blythe, J. G., Prophylactic chemotherapy in stage I and II uterine sarcoma. *Gynecologic Oncology*, 1979, **8**, 346–8.

Christopherson, W. M., Williamson, E. O., Gray, L. A., Leiomyosarcoma of the uterus. *Cancer*, 1972, **29**, 1512–17.

Creagan, E. T., Hahn, R. G., Ahmann, D. L., Edmonson, J. H., Bisel, H. F., Eagan, R. T., A comparative trial evaluating the combination of adriamycin, DTIC and vincristine, the combination of actinomycin D, cyclophosphamide and vincristine and a single agent methylCCNU in advanced sarcomas. *Cancer Treat. Rep.*, 1976, **60**, 1385.

Giuliano, A. E., Larkin, K. L., Silber, F. R., Morton, D. L., Failure of combination chemotherapy (CYVADIC) in metastatic soft tissue sarcoma: implication for adjuvant studies. *Proc. Am. Assoc. Cancer Res. and ASCO*, 1978, **18**, 359.

Gottlieb, J. A., Baker, L. H., Quagliana, J. M., Luce, J. K., Whitecar, J. P., Sinkovics, J. G., Rivlin, S. E., Brownlee, R., Frei, E. III, Chemotherapy of sarcomas with combinations of adriamycin and dimethyltriazene—imidazole carboxamide. *Cancer*, 1972, **30**, 1632–8.

Gottlieb, J. A., Bodey, G. P., Sinkovics, J. G., et al., An effective new 4-drug combination regimen (CY-VA-DIC) for metastatic sarcomas. *Proc. Am. Assoc. Cancer Res. and ASCO*, 1974, **15**, 162.

Hart, W. R., Billman, J. K., Jr., A reassessment of uterine neoplasms originally diagnosed as leiomyosarcoma. *Cancer*, 1978, **41**, 1902–10.

Karakousis, C. P., Holtermann, O. A., Holyoke, E. D., Cisdichlorodiammine platinum (II) in metastatic soft tissue sarcoma. *Cancer Treat. Rep.*, 1979, **63**, 2071–5.

Kempson, R. L., Bari, W., Uterine sarcoma: classification, diagnosis and prognosis. *Hum. Pathol.*, 1970, **1**, 331–49.

Krumholz, B. A., Lobovsky, F. Y., Halitsky, V., Endolyphatic stromal myosis with pulmonary metastases—remission with progestin therapy. *J. Reprod. Med.*, 1973, **10**, 85–9.

Lehrner, L. M., Miles, P. A., Enck, R. E., Complete remission of widely metastatic endometrial stromal carcinoma following combination chemotherapy. *Cancer*, 1979, **43**, 1189–94.

Montague, A. C. W., Swartz, D. P., Woodruff, J. O., Sarcoma arising in a leiomyoma of uterus. *Am. J. Obstet. Gynecol.*, 1965, **92**, 421–7.

Novak, E., Anderson, D. F., Sarcoma of the uterus. *Am. J. Obstet. Gynecol.*, 1937, **34**, 740–61.

Omura, G. A., Shingleton, H. M., Creasman, W. T., Blessing, J. A., Boronow, R. C., Chemotherapy of gynecologic cancer with nitrosoureas: a randomised trial of CCNU and methyl CCNU in cancers of the cervix, corpus, vagina and vulva. *Cancer Treat. Rep.*, 1978a, **62**, 833.

Omura, G. A., Blessing, J. A., Chemotherapy of stage III, IV and recurrent uterine sarcoma: a randomised trial of adriamycin versus adriamycin and dimethyl triazeno imidazol carboxamide (DTIC), *Amer. Assoc. Cancer Res. and ASCO*, 1978b, **19**, 26.

Parente, J. T., Axelrod, M. R., Levy, J. L., Chiang, C. E., Leiomyosarcoma of the uterus with pulmonary metastases: A favourable response to operation and chemotherapy in a patient monitored with serial carcinoembryonic antigen. *Am. J. Obstet. Gynecol.*, 1978, **131** (7), 812–15.

Piver, M. S., Barlow, J. J., Lele, S. B., Yazigi, R., Adriamycin in localised and metastatic uterine sarcomas. *J. Surg. Oncol.*, 1979, **12** (3), 263–5.

Piver, M. S., Lurain, J. R., Uterine sarcomas: clinical features and management in: *Gynecologic Oncology*, ed. Coppleson, M., Churchill Livingstone, 1981, pp. 615–16.

Rosenbaum, C., Schoenfield, D., Treatment of advanced soft tissue sarcoma. *Proc. Am. Soc. Clin. Oncol.*, 1977, **18**, 287.

Smith, J. P., Rutledge, F., Advances in chemotherapy for gynecologic cancer. *Cancer*, 1975a, **36**, 669–74.

Smith, J. P., Rutledge, F., Declos, L., Sutow, W., Combined irradiation and chemotherapy for sarcomas of the pelvis in females. *Am. J. Roentgenol. Rad. Ther. Nucl. Med.*, 1975b, **123**, 571.

Smith, J. R., Sarcoma of uterus. *New York State J. Med.*, 1941, **41**, 681.

Subraminian, S., Wiltshaw, E., Chemotherapy for sarcomas. *Lancet*, 1978, **1**, 683–6.

Thigpen, J. T., Shingleton, H., Homesley, H., DiSaia, P., Lagasse, L., Blessing, J. In *Cisplatin: current status and new developments*. ed. Prestayko, A. W., Crooke, S. T., Carter, S. K. Academic Press Inc., New York, 1980, p. 416.

Yazigi, R., Piver, M. S., Barlow, J. J., Stage III uterine sarcoma: case report and literature review. *Gynecologic Oncology*, 1979, **8**, 92–96.

Yoonessi, M., Hart, W. R., Endometrial stromal sarcomas. *Cancer*, 1977, **40**, 898–906.

Chapter Twenty One

Genital Rhabdomyosarcoma—Sarcoma Botryoides

Vaginal and uterine rhabdomyosarcomas, also known as mixed mesodermal tumours, are rare—only 13 were seen at the Memorial Center for Cancer, New York, between 1939 and 1958 (Daniel 1959). Early diagnosis is of prognostic importance but delays in diagnosis are unfortunately common; Daniel (1959) reported such a delay of up to four years in some of his reported cases. Hoffman (1981) cautions that although sarcoma botryoides is rare, anything resembling it clinically, eg 'proud flesh', 'fibromatous polyp', is rarer still.

They usually appear in the first six to eighteen months of life, and occasionally as late as early adulthood. The primary lesion frequently arises from the anterior wall of the vagina adjacent to, or apparently arising from, the cervix. It may also be in the distal vagina or labia (Sutow et al. 1970). Guérsant and Wagner are independently credited with the first description of these tumours in 1854, although it was Pfannenstiel, in 1892, who coined the term sarcoma botryoides. However, some of these tumours do not have a grape-like appearance.

Bladder neck invasion is much more common than invasion of the rectum. Lymph nodal or extrapelvic spread is infrequent. Limited surgical excision is nearly always followed by recurrence (Ortega et al. 1975). Four patients treated at the Memorial Center for Cancer, New York, during the 1950s by only hysterectomy and vaginectomy all perished within 20 months (Hilgers et al. 1973).

Successful treatment of a proportion of children is offered by pelvic exenteration followed by radical radiotherapy. The use of chemotherapy, eg VAC (vincristine, actinomycin D and cyclophosphamide) has improved survival markedly, and three year disease free survival rates have been reported as 60–90% in Los Angeles (Hay 1980).

However, a high price is paid in terms of post-therapy morbidity—urinary bypass, stomas, infertility and impotence. Attempts are now being made to reduce this morbidity by reducing the extent of necessary surgery by initial chemotherapy with VAC (Tank et al. 1972), possibly omitting the irradiation and continuing chemotherapy for a further two years.

Chemosensitivity of these tumours is commonly found and survival rates with limited surgery (simple hysterectomy and partial vaginectomy) combined with

Table 21.1   Chemotherapy of genital rhabdomyosarcoma

Source	Age of patient	Site	Chemotherapy	Tumour-free survival (months)
Heyn (1974)	3 years	Vagina	VCR + ACTD	79+
	11 months	Vagina	VCR + ACTD	47+
Ghavimi (1975)	1 year	Uterus	VCR + ACTD + ADRIA + CYCLO	33+
	12 years	Uterus	VCR + ACTD + ADRIA + CYCLO	15+
Kumar (1976)	8 months	Vagina	VCR + ACTD + CYCLO	44+
	11 years	Vagina	VCR + ACTD + CYCLO	32+
	17 years	Uterus	VCR + ACTD + CYCLO	54+

VCR = vincristine, ACTD = actinomycin D, ADRIA = adriamycin, CYCLO = cyclophosphamide

chemotherapy have been excellent. Kumar et al. (1976), reported tumour free continuing survival of girls so treated at 32, 44 and 54 months with no appreciable alteration in the quality of life and planned vaginoplasty during adulthood; see Table 21.1.

Exelby et al. (1978) report the use of additional agents to the established VAC regimen such as bleomycin, adriamycin and methotrexate.

It now seems reasonable to treat these tumours initially with VAC and to perform limited surgery when tumour shrinkage has been produced and to continue chemotherapy for one to two years reserving radical surgery (eg anterior exenteration) for those tumours not responding to initial VAC within the first few months of treatment.

References

Daniel, W., Sarcoma botryoides of the vagina. *Cancer*, 1959, **12**, 74.

Exelby, P. R., Ghavimi, F., Jereb, B., Genitourinary rhabdomyosarcoma in children. *J. Paediatr. Surg.*, 1978, **13**, 746–52.

Hay, D. M., Pelvic rhabdomyosarcomas in childhood. *Cancer*, 1980, **45**, 1810–14.

Heyn, R., Holland, R., Newton, W., Tefft, M., Breslow, N., Hartmann, J. R., The role of combined therapy in the treatment of rhabdomyosarcoma in children. *Cancer*, 1974, **34**, 2128–42.

Hilgers, R. D., Ghavimi, F., D'Angio, G. J., Exelby, P., Lewis, J. L., Memorial Hospital experience with pelvic exenteration and embryonal rhabdomyosarcoma of the vagina. *Gynecologic Oncology*, 1973, **1**, 262–70.

Ghavimi, F., Exelby, P. R., D'Angio, G. J. et al., Multidisciplinary treatment of embryonal rhabdomyosarcomas in children. *Cancer*, 1975, **35**, 677–86.

Guérsant, P., Polypes du vagin chez une petite fille de treize mois. *Moniteur Hôpiteaux*, 1854, **2**, 187.

Hoffman, J. W., *The gynecology of childhood and adolescence*. W. B. Saunders, 1981, pp. 253, 268.

Kumar, A., Wrenn, E. L., Fleming, I. D., Hustu, H. O., Pratt, C. B., Combined therapy to prevent complete pelvic exenteration for rhabdomyosarcoma of the vagina and uterus. *Cancer*, 1976, **37**, 118–22.

Ortega, J. A., Rivard, G., Hittle, R. E., Karon, M. R., Hays, D. M., Limited surgery in the management of pelvic rhabdomyosarcoma. In proceedings of a symposium: *Conflicts in childhood cancer*, Roswell Park Memorial Institute, 1975, 375–84.

Pfannenstiel, J., Das traubige sarcom der cervix uteri. *Virchows Arch. (Pathol. Anat.)*, 1892, **127**, 305.

Sutow, W. W., Sullivan, M. P., Reid, H. L., Taylor, H. G., Griffith, K. M., Prognosis in childhood rhabdomyosarcoma. *Cancer*, 1970, **25**, 1384–90.

Tank, E. S., Fellmann, S. L., Wheeler, E. S., Weaver, D. K., Lapides, J., Treatment of urogenital tract rhabdomyosarcoma in infants and children. *J. Urol.*, 1972, **107**, 324–8.

Wagner, E. (quoted by Pfannenstiel, 1892), Mixed mesodermal tumor of uterus—first description, 1854.

Chapter Twenty Two

Future Prospects

The future prospects for the management of gynaecological cancers and other solid tumours must be regarded with controlled optimism. A better understanding of the aetiology and biology of the malignant processes involved will enable more effective forms of therapy to be developed. Improvements in knowledge concerning the immunological reactions which do, and do not, take place when tumours appear may also lead to further means of destroying them. More integrated and varied applications of the existing anticancer modalities, eg giving chemotherapy before radiotherapy or surgery, may also increase cure rates.

Diagnosis at an early stage of the disease is always of prognostic significance. However, despite screening systems and campaigns in various countries, the goal of prevention or early diagnosis of all gynaecological cancers is still remote. Nine out of ten women presenting with invasive carcinoma of the cervix in the UK have never had a Papanicolaou smear. The establishment of pelvic ultrasound surveillance research units in London may yield some information about the natural history of ovarian cancer (of which there is insufficient knowledge) in postmenopausal women, and possibly offer a means of early diagnosis. The practical problems of operating such a system on a widespread scale are considerable.

The discovery of reliable tumour markers detectable in the peripheral blood stream at a very early stage may offer a simple, practical method of screening populations at risk which could be carried out on a large scale.

Dr Ion Gresser in France first suggested in the 1960s that virally induced tumours may be affected by the administration of the antiviral protein interferon—first identified by Isaacs and Lindenmann in London in 1957. Interferon was subsequently shown to arrest the division of tumour cells in vitro; and later in vivo including those cells which were thought to be resistant to interferon in vitro. Interferon may therefore act by stimulating the host defence systems, possibly by alteration of the tumour cell membrane characteristics and increasing its antigencity. Clinical temporary tumour remissions have been observed using interferon and the use of regimens combining cytotoxic drugs with interferon are being investigated (Priestman 1980, Scott and Tyrell 1980, Sikora 1980).

The current developments in chemotherapy can be broadly divided into two groups: (1) improvement in the use of drugs available now and (2) the development of new cytotoxic agents.

Improved use of existing agents

Increasing the dose

It has often been suggested that 'small doses of chemotherapy produce responses whereas big doses produce remissions' and that so-called cytotoxic agent resistance' in a tumour, or lack of drug responsiveness, is really only a dose relationship which has not been increased sufficiently to produce a response. Whereas that may not be totally true, it should now be obvious that unless sufficient agent is used to eliminate all the stem cells of a tumour, then a cure is not possible.

But increasing drug doses also means increasing side effects and toxicity. Ways of avoiding this are being sought. Workers at the Royal Marsden Hospital, Surrey, England, have been able to give large doses of an alkylating agent using autologous marrow grafting and gut protection with low dose cyclophosphamide pretreatment. Millar et al. (1978) showed that the intestinal epithelium of mice and sheep receiving large doses of melphalan (thought to be a good stem cell poison) could receive considerable protection from the expected desquamation (see page 16) and that similar cyclophosphamide pretreatment could accelerate bone marrow recovery in humans receiving high dose melphalan therapy (Hedley et al. 1978). The half-life of melphalan is about one hour; most is excreted from the body within six hours. Cyclophosphamide 'priming' is given one week before to protect the gut and halve the neutropoenia time. Diarrhoea is produced using 170 mg/m^2 without priming, or at 260 mg/m^2 after priming. Bone marrow is aspirated from the patient in the morning, the very large dose of melphalan is given and the marrow returned to the patient from cryopreservation via an intravenous drip some 12 hours later, when nearly all the melphalan has been excreted.

It is hoped that having demonstrated drug sensitivity in patients with ovarian carcinoma they could then enter immediate and prolonged remission using high dose alkylating agent therapy. Harper and Souhami, at University College Hospital, London, operate a similar system with very high dose cyclophosphamide, with other agents to protect the bladder epithelium.

Increasing selectivity

Higher concentration of cytotoxic agents in tumours than in normal tissues may also be achieved by joining the agent onto a substance which is selectively absorbed by the tumour. Chapter 5 gave a list of those substances secreted by tumours—it is possible that antibodies (eg monoclonal) to the tumour cell surface protein may be suitable for targeting cytotoxic agents and the use of liposomes to contain these 'letter bombs' is being explored.

Antibodies to tumour markers, eg beta subunit of HCG, and alphafetoprotein, may also be of therapeutic value and are being developed, along with hormones taken up selectively by tumours, to be attached to cytotoxics. There is some evidence to suggest that antibodies against target tumour antigens, without cytotoxic agents, may be able to attack specific malignancies (Trowbridge and Domingo 1981).

Harris and his colleagues in Oxford, UK (1982), have discovered a new marker substance in tumour cell surfaces called Ca antigen. Using monoclonal antibodies and radioimmunoassay, antibody Ca1 was produced and was found to bind to the membranes of cervical carcinoma cells but not to normal cells, except those of the fallopian tube epithelium and bladder. The possible conjugation of the antibody with cytotoxic agents is being explored.

Administration and schedule variation

Despite the lack of widespread success in attempting to apply cell kinetic theories to the scheduling of chemotherapy (Bush 1979) thought is being given to administering cytotoxic agents in less traditional ways, eg comparing bolus injections with infusions, and varying dose interval times. Dose limiting toxicity and side effects may well be reduced allowing higher drug tolerance and, it is hoped, increasing cell kill.

There is some evidence that the toxicity of doxorubicin (adriamycin) may well be reduced by administering the agent in small weekly doses rather than in larger monthly ones. Evidence is also being accumulated to show that the scheduling of etoposide (VP16) affects its efficacy considerably. The assessment of new agents in clinical trials now takes account of scheduling variations in order to discover their full potential.

Analogues of existing agents

Much research effort is devoted to produce analogues of existing cytotoxic agents with similar modes of action but greater efficacy and/or less toxicity and side effects. Structure-activity relationships are examined and similar compounds are produced and then screened for cytotoxic activity. An example of this approach is the large number of platinum complexes (in excess of 500) which have been synthesised and investigated for antitumour activity—mainly based upon the PtX_2A_2 (X_2 = two monodentate, or one bidentate anionic ligands; A_2 = two monodentate, or one bidentate amine ligands) complex (Cleare et al. 1980). Approximately, half a dozen compounds have been selected for clinical trials. One such compound JM8 (1,1-cyclobutanedicarboxylate diammineplatinum II = $Pt(NH_3)_2CBDCA$) is hoped to be as effective as cisplatin but much less myelotoxic and nephrotoxic, and is currently under clinical evaluation at the Royal Marsden Hospital, London.

JM8

Development of new cytotoxic agents

'The proper study of mankind is man'
Alexander Pope (1688–1744) An Essay On Man, Epistle ii, 1.2.

Between 1966 and 1975, 264 000 chemicals were screened by the National Cancer Institute and only 132 of these agents showed sufficient cytotoxic effect in mice to proceed to large animal toxicology studies and clinical trials (Tattersall 1981).

Commonly, the L1210 leukaemia induced in mice (with 3-methylcholanthrene) is used as the main tumour model against which new substances are screened for antitumour activity. Toxicities are evaluated using a variety of doses given to dogs. Lethality and toxicity may also be evaluated in monkeys. Phase One and Two studies are then performed with selected compounds—see Chapter 4, page 18, and finally, phase three studies compare the new agents against established treatment. Before widespread marketed use toxicology and other requirements of the national regulatory bodies, eg Committee for the Safety of Medicines (UK), and the Federal Drugs Administration (USA), must be fulfilled.

Concern has recently been expressed concerning the value and effectiveness of such new compound screening. Principal points of anxiety are:

(a) the length of time the above studies take, not to mention the cost. If the cure for cancer was in the laboratory of today it would be at least a decade before the compound was in widespread use. Toxicology animal screening itself takes about two years.

(b) are mouse leukaemia tumours the best models on which to test drugs likely to be effective against human tumours? Several compounds which were initially rejected have later been shown to have activity in other systems.

(c) is the toxicology screen necessary beyond the mouse? Dogs, for example, offer a good model for gastrointestinal effects but there is poor correlation between renal and hepatic effects in dogs and humans.

(d) should agents proceed to Phase One clinical trials earlier—after all, the human tumour in humans is the ideal, and signs of early toxicity of new compounds may be detected by clinicians in carefully controlled situations.

Some of these problems are accommodated by the recent inclusion of other in vitro and in vivo testing systems in alternative screening processes, eg xenografted tumours. The current National Cancer Institute Drug Development programme attempts to screen about 500–1000 new compounds each year and reduces the number submitted with a pre-screen using the mouse leukaemia P388 tumour model as shown in Figure 22.1 (Goldin et al. 1979, Venditti 1982).

Demonstrably active compounds are now being evaluated relatively speedily by coordinating the clinical studies in computer linked centres with the NCI in the USA and via the New Drugs Development Coordinating Committee of the EORTC in Europe.

New cytotoxic agents are emerging. Industry has provided several active groups of substances. Mitoxantrone and bisantrene, from the anthracendione group of dyestuffs, are being evaluated (Cornbleet and Smyth 1982) after showing activity in a variety of human tumours. Produced in Japan, aclacynomycin appears to be

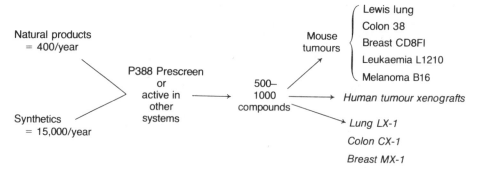

Fig. 22.1 National Cancer Institute new compound screen

similar to doxorubicin (adriamycin) but causing no alopecia and much less cardio-toxicity. Again from industry some compounds used in washing powders are being evaluated, and from ball-point pen ink comes an anthracene called ametantrone which has reached phase I studies in the USA. Trope (1981) has reported phase II studies in Sweden of spirogermanium, which belongs to the azaspiranes, and has been shown to inhibit protein synthesis in vitro and to have a cytotoxic effect on HeLa cells and Walker 256 carcinosarcoma. Out of 18 heavily pretreated patients with advanced ovarian carcinoma treated with spirogermanium, two patients had objective responses (duration 5 and 23+ months) and 4 had stable disease. There were few side effects.

It is hoped that current production and screening methods will deliver new active cytotoxic agents into the hands of clinicians as quickly as possible within the limits of safety—it therefore behoves clinicians to apply themselves to the problem of administering these agents to their patients by the most compassionate and efficacious means possible.

References

Bush, R. S. *Malignancies of the ovary, uterus and cervix.* Edward Arnold, 1979, pp. 227–8.

Cleare, M. J., Hydes, P. C., Hepburn, D. R., Malerbi, B. W., Antitumour platinum complexes: Structure-activity relationships. In: *Cisplatin: current status and new developments.* Ed. Prestayko, A. W., Crooke, S. T., Carter, S. K., Academic Press, New York, 1980, pp. 149–70.

Cornbleet, M. A., Smyth, J. F., Report of the ASCO/AACR symposium 1982. *Cancer Topics,* **4**, No. 1, July/August 1982, p. 10.

Goldin, A., Schepartz, S. A., Venditti, J. M., De Vita, V. T. In: *Methods of Cancer Research, Vol. XVI,* Academic Press, New York, 1979, p. 165.

Harris, D. L., Ashall, F., Bramwell, M. E., McGee, J. O'D., Woods, J. C., A new marker for human cancer cells Parts I and II. *Lancet,* 1982, **ii**, 1–10.

Hedley, D. W., McElwain, T. J., Millar, J. L., Gordon, M. J., Acceleration of bone marrow recovery by pretreatment with cyclophosphamide to patients receiving high dose melphalan. *Lancet,* 1978, **2**, 966.

Millar, J. L., Husdpith, B. N., McElwain, T. J., Phelps, T. A., Effect of high dose melphalan on marrow and intestinal epithelium in mice pre-treated with cyclo-phosphamide. *Br. J. Cancer,* 1978, **38**, 137.

Priestman, T. J., Initial evaluation of human lymphoblastoid interferon in patients with advanced malignant disease. *Lancet*, 1980, **2**, 113–18.

Scott, G. M., Tyrell, D. A. J., Interferon: therapeutic fact or fiction for the 80s? *Br. Med. J.*, 1980, **i**, 1558–62.

Sikora, K., Does interferon cure cancer? *Br. Med. J.*, 1980, **ii**, 885–8.

Tattersall, M. H. N., In *Gynecologic Oncology: principles and clinical practice Vol. 1.*, ed. Coppelson M., Churchill Livingstone, Edinburgh, 1981, p. 121.

Trope, C., Mattsson, W., Gynning, I., Johnson, J.-E., Sigurdsson, K., Orbert, B., Phase II study of spirogermanium in advanced ovarian malignancy. *Cancer Treat. Rep.*, 1981, **65**, 119–20.

Trowbridge, I. S., Domingo, D. L., Anti-transferrin receptor monoclonal antibody and toxin-antibody conjugates effect growth of human tumour cells. *Nature*, 1981, **294**, 171–3.

Venditti, J. M., The Model's Dilemma, in *Design of Models for Testing Cancer Therapeutic Agents*, ed. Fidler, I. J., White, R. J., Von Nostrand Reinhold Co., New York, 1982, pp. 80–94.

Index

145